Clinical Controversies in Device Therapy for Cardiac Arrhythmias

Jonathan S. Steinberg • Andrew E. Epstein
Editors

Clinical Controversies in Device Therapy for Cardiac Arrhythmias

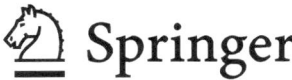 Springer

Editors
Jonathan S. Steinberg
University of Rochester
School of Medicine &
Dentistry/Hackensack Meridian
School of Medicine at Seton Hall
University/Summit Medical Group
Short Hills
NJ, USA

Andrew E. Epstein
Electrophysiology Section, Cardiovascular
Division
Univeristy of Pennsylvania, and
the Cardiology Division
Corporal Michael J. Crescenz VA Medical
Center
Philadelphia
PA, USA

ISBN 978-3-030-22881-1   ISBN 978-3-030-22882-8   (eBook)
https://doi.org/10.1007/978-3-030-22882-8

This Springer imprint is published by the registered company Springer Nature Switzerland AG
The registered company address is: Gewerbestrasse 11, 6330 Cham, Switzerland

Preface

The treatment of patients with and at risk for bradycardia, tachycardia, and heart failure depends on implantable and wearable cardiac electrical devices. Cardiac implantable electrical devices (CIEDs) include pacemakers, implantable cardioverter-defibrillators, cardiac resynchronization devices, and implantable monitors. CIEDs are managed by a variety of health-care providers including electrophysiologists, cardiologists, and associated professionals including nurses and technicians.

Many management issues for patients with CIEDs are well established and straightforward. Others are more complex and challenging and have a body of published medical evidence that is ambiguous, poorly defined, or controversial.

This book addresses the most important of the tough contemporary clinical issues facing clinical cardiac electrophysiology providers and is designed to support those who treat patients in real-world practice. It includes contributions by widely recognized international leaders in the field and focuses on the most unsettled controversies. Genuine experts have been charged with creating practical value to clinicians and staff members. High-profile and sometimes controversial contemporary topics include implantable defibrillators for nonischemic cardiomyopathy, His-bundle pacing, ethical issues at end life, risk stratification, decision-making for resynchronization devices, and much more.

Short Hills, NJ, USA   Jonathan S. Steinberg
Philadelphia, PA, USA   Andrew E. Epstein

Contents

Contributors

Selcuk Adabag Cardiology Division, Minneapolis Veterans Affairs Health Care System, Minneapolis, MN, USA

Division of Cardiology, Department of Medicine, Cardiology (111C), Minneapolis, MN, USA

Department of Cardiovascular Medicine, University of Minnesota, Minneapolis, MN, USA

Evan Adelstein Albany Medical College, Albany, NY, USA

Vidhu Anand Department of Cardiovascular Medicine, Mayo Clinic, Rochester, MN, USA

K. Dickstein Institute of Internal Medicine, University of Bergen, Bergen, Norway

Cardiology Division, Stavanger University Hospital, Stavanger, Norway

Alejandra Gutierrez Department of Cardiovascular Medicine, University of Minnesota, Minneapolis, MN, USA

Nicole Habel University of Vermont Medical Center, Burlington, VT, USA

Lars Køber The Heart Centre, Rigshospitalet, University of Copenhagen, Copenhagen, Denmark

Valentina Kutyifa Clinical Cardiovascular Research Center, Cardiology Division, University of Rochester Medical Center, Rochester, NY, USA

Rachel Lampert Yale University School of Medicine, New Haven, CT, USA

Francisco Leyva Aston Medical Research Institute, Aston Medical School, Aston University, Birmingham, UK

Daniel L. Lustgarten University of Vermont Medical Center, Burlington, VT, USA

C. Normand Cardiology Division, Stavanger University Hospital, Stavanger, Norway

Institute of Internal Medicine, University of Bergen, Bergen, Norway

Christopher Piorkowski Heart Center Dresden University Hospital, Department of Invasive Electrophysiology, Dresden, Germany

Samir Saba Heart and Vascular Institute, University of Pittsburgh Medical Center, Pittsburgh, PA, USA

Martin Stockburger Havelland Kliniken, Academic Teaching Hospital of Charité – Universitaetsmedizin Berlin, Nauen, Germany

Jens Jakob Thune Department of Cardiology, Bispebjerg and Frederiksberg Hospital, University of Copenhagen, Copenhagen, Denmark

Jakub Tomala Heart Center Dresden University Hospital, Department of Invasive Electrophysiology, Dresden, Germany

Roderick Tung Center for Arrhythmia Care, Heart and Vascular Institute, University of Chicago Medicine, The Pritzker School of Medicine at the University of Chicago, Chicago, IL, USA

Gaurav A. Upadhyay Center for Arrhythmia Care, Heart and Vascular Institute, University of Chicago Medicine, The Pritzker School of Medicine at the University of Chicago, Chicago, IL, USA

Norman Wang Heart and Vascular Institute, University of Pittsburgh Medical Center, Pittsburgh, PA, USA

Hannah E. Wey Department of Internal Medicine, University of Chicago Medicine, The Pritzker School of Medicine at the University of Chicago, Chicago, IL, USA

Chapter 1
The Use of Implantable Cardioverter-Defibrillators in Nonischemic Cardiomyopathy

Jens Jakob Thune and Lars Køber

Introduction

In people with cardiac arrest due to ventricular arrhythmia, the application of an electrical shock to the myocardium may terminate the ventricular arrhythmia and resuscitate the patient. In 1985, the approval of the implantable cardioverter-defibrillator made it possible to protect persons at high risk of cardiac arrest. While the first versions of the ICD were bulky and had to be placed in the abdomen with epicardial shock wires placed surgically, improvements in the design has made ICD implantation no more complicated than conventional pacemaker placement. Hence, ICDs today may be implanted in almost any patient and the decision to implant an ICD is based on an assessment of the likelihood of obtaining lifesaving therapy from the device compared to the short- and long-term risks associated with implantation, such as infection and inappropriate shocks.

Nonischemic cardiomyopathy is an umbrella term for a wide array of myocardial diseases where the impaired myocardial function is not caused by coronary artery disease. Thus, nonischemic cardiomyopathy may be secondary to valvular heart disease, congenital heart disease, or hypertension; it may be part of a systemic disease such as sarcoidosis, systemic lupus, or amyloidosis; it may be genetic such as hypertrophic cardiomyopathy, arrhythmogenic ventricular cardiomyopathy, or familial dilated cardiomyopathy; it may be caused by drugs such as cocaine or antineoplastic compounds; it may be caused by infection; or it may be idiopathic.

J. J. Thune (✉)
Department of Cardiology, Bispebjerg and Frederiksberg Hospital,
University of Copenhagen, Copenhagen, Denmark
e-mail: jjt@heart.dk

L. Køber
The Heart Centre, Rigshospitalet, University of Copenhagen, Copenhagen, Denmark
e-mail: Lars.Koeber.01@regionh.dk

© Springer Nature Switzerland AG 2019
J. S. Steinberg, A. E. Epstein (eds.), *Clinical Controversies in Device Therapy for Cardiac Arrhythmias*, https://doi.org/10.1007/978-3-030-22882-8_1

This chapter discusses the use of ICDs in patients with heart failure and reduced left ventricle systolic function, which is not explained by coronary artery disease.

Secondary Prevention

As ICDs work by terminating malignant ventricular arrhythmia, the persons most likely to benefit are those who have already had such an arrythmia. Therefore, ICDs are offered to everyone with nonischemic cardiomyopathy, who have had ventricular fibrillation or sustained ventricular tachycardia, where the arrythmia was not due to obviously reversible factors such as severe hypokalemia, or the patient has a very high risk of death within a year due to other causes.

Three secondary prevention trials included a combined 292 patients with non-ischemic cardiomyopathy, the Antiarrhythmics versus Implantable Defibrillators Trial (AVID) [1], the Canadian Implantable Defibrillator Study CIDS) [2], and the Cardiac Arrest Study Hamburg (CASH) [3]. Of these trials, only AVID and CIDS reported outcomes for the subgroup of patients with nonischemic cardiomyopathy. Both trials found a trend towards reduction in mortality with ICD implantation, but because of the low number of patients, neither was statistically significant. In a combined analysis of the two trials, ICD implantation was associated with a hazard ratio of 0.69 with a statistically nonsignificant p-value of 0.22 [4]. However, when including the much larger number of patients with ischemic heart disease in the analysis, the reduction in mortality becomes statistically significant and with no hint of a difference in effect of ICD implantation between patients with and without ischemic heart disease [5]. For this reason, guidelines recommend that all patients who have survived a sustained ventricular arrhythmia should be offered an ICD.

Primary Prevention

Some patients with nonischemic systolic heart failure are at such high risk of death due to ventricular arrhythmia that an ICD is recommended for primary prevention. However, the risk of sudden cardiac is lower than for patients who have already experienced arrhythmia. This means that other competing causes of death become relatively more likely and that the survival benefit from an ICD decreases while the risk of complications is unchanged.

There have been six primary prevention trials in which patients with nonischemic cardiomyopathy were included, Table 1.1.

The trials were comparable in some respects such as the typical patient being a middle-aged Caucasian male with severely reduced left ventricular ejection fraction. But because trials were conducted over a 15-year period, there was a marked

Table 1.1   Trials of ICD implantation for primary prevention including patients with nonsichemic cardiomyopathy

	CAT [6]	AMIOVIRT [7]	DEFINITE [8]	SCD-HeFT[a] [9]	COMPANION[b] [10]	DANISH [11]
Number of patients in trial	104	103	458	2521	1520	1117
Number of patients in ICD arm	50	51	229	829	595	557
Age (years)	52 (mean)	59 (mean)	58 (mean)	60	66	63
Nonischemic etiology	100	100	100	48	45	100
Male	80	71	71	77	67	72
Duration of heart failure	3 months (mean)	3.2 years (mean)	2.8 years (mean)	NR	3.5 years	1.8 years
CRT	–	–	–	–	100 [c]	58
Atrial fibrillation	16	NR	25	17	0	22
Diabetes	NR	34	23	31	41	19
LVEF	24 (mean)	23	21 (mean)	24	22	25
QRS (ms)	108 (mean)	NR	112ms (mean)	NR	160	146
NYHA						
I		15	22	–	–	–
II	65	63	57	68	–	54
III	35	20	21	32	86	45
IV			–	–	14	1
Medication						
ACE/ARB	96	85	86–97	94	90	97
Beta blocker	4	51	85	69	68	92
MRA	NR	19	NR	20	55	58
Follow-up time (months)	66 (mean)	24 (mean)	29 (mean)	46	16	68

Numbers represent percent or median unless indicated
ARB angiotensin receptor blocker, *MRA* mineralocorticoid receptor antagonist, *CRT* cardiac resynchronization therapy, *CAT* the cardiomyopathy trial, *AMIOVIRT* amiodarone versus implantable cardioverter-defibrillator: randomized trial in patients with nonischemic dilated cardiomyopathy and asymptomatic nonsustained ventricular tachycardia, *DEFINITE* defibrillators in nonischemic cardiomyopathy treatment evaluation, *NR* not reported, *SCD-HeFT* sudden cardiac death in heart failure trial, *COMPANION* comparison of medical therapy, pacing, and defibrillation in heart failure, *DANISH* Danish study to assess the efficacy of ICDs in patients with nonischemic systolic heart failure on mortality
[a]Descriptive statistics are presented for the ICD group ($n = 829$)
[b]Descriptive statistics are presented for the CRT-D group ($n = 595$)
[c]No patients received an ICD only, patients who got a device received cardiac resynchronization therapy with or without a defibrillator

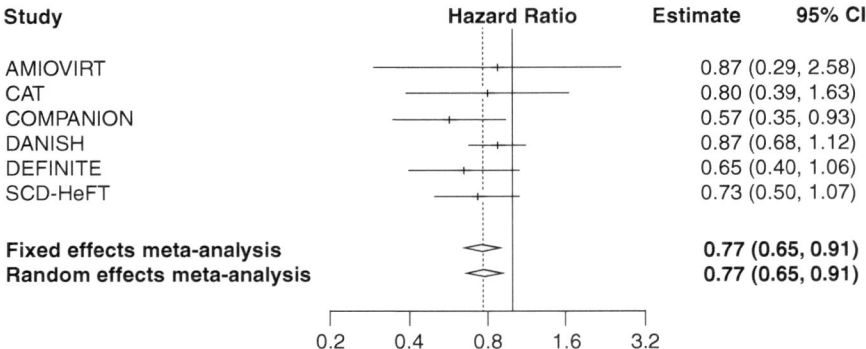

Fig. 1.1 Meta-analysis of the effect of ICD-implantation on all-cause death in patients with non-sichemic cardiomyopathy. lower hazard ratio favors ICDw

difference in concomitant medical therapy, and consequently a wide difference in risk of all-cause and sudden cardiac death. Most of the trials had fewer patients on betablockers and mineralocorticoid receptor antagonist than would be acceptable with current medical management of heart failure patients. Four trials included only patients with nonischemic heart failure, while the two remaining trials included both patients with ischemic and nonischemic etiology.

Only DEFINITE and DANISH were designed and powered to detect a difference in all-cause mortality for patients with nonischemic heart failure. Both trials were neutral. The SCD-HeFT trial did not specifically find a p-value below 0.05 in the subgroup of patients with nonischemic heart failure, but this was very likely due to low power as there was no interaction between ischemic or nonischemic etiology on the effect of ICD implantation. The only trial with a p-value below 0.05 for the effect of ICD implantation in patients with nonischemic heart failure was the post hoc comparison of patients with nonischemic etiology who received cardiac resynchronization therapy with or without a defibrillator function in COMPANION. Yet, all trials trended towards a mortality lowering effect of ICD implantation, and taken together there is a statistically significant 23% reduction in hazard of all-cause death with ICD implantation (Fig. 1.1). This reduction in all-cause mortality is driven by a substantial 60% reduction in sudden cardiac death. Because of these results, international guidelines recommend ICD implantation in patients with nonischemic systolic heart failure [12, 13].

Individual Risk Stratification

For some patients with nonischemic systolic heart failure, an ICD is not likely to substantially prolong life. This is the case for patients who are either simply at a low risk of sudden cardiac death in general or patients with a nonnegligible risk of sudden cardiac death but whose risk of death from nonsudden causes overshadows this risk. For such patients, the risk-benefit ratio with ICD implantation is reduced.

Age-specific treatment effect

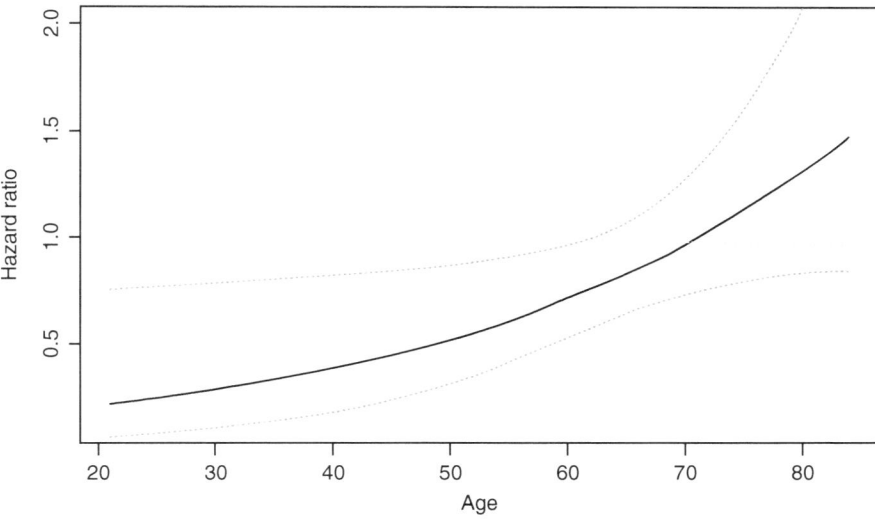

Fig. 1.2 The relation between age and risk of all-cause mortality regarding ICD treatment or control. On the x-axis age in years and on the y-axis the hazard ratio (HR). The dashed blue line indicates hazard ratio =1, which corresponds to an equal mortality in patients treated with ICD and control. The black line illustrates the risk for all-cause mortality according to age, and the dashed red lines are the 95% confidence interval. ICD denotes implantable cardioverter-defibrillator

An example of this is older patients. In the DANISH trial, there was a significant interaction between the age and the effect of ICD implantation on all-cause mortality in that older patients did not benefit from ICD implantation as opposed to younger patients (Fig. 1.2) [14]. This decline in effect of ICD implantation with age was due to a decrease in relative risk of sudden cardiac death compared to other modes of death with age. While the absolute risk of sudden cardiac death was unchanged in older patients, the risk of nonsudden death was markedly increased. And as ICD implantation only affects sudden cardiac death, the benefit of ICD implantation decreased, not because of a reduced effect on sudden cardiac death, but because of a much higher risk of other modes of death.

In line with this thinking, investigators attempt to identify patients at high absolute and relative risk of sudden cardiac death. It does remain, however, very difficult to identify risk factors that increase the risk of dying suddenly as opposed to dying nonsuddenly, as most risk factors increase the risk of both sudden and nonsudden death equally. The Seattle Proportional Risk Model was developed to determine the likelihood of death being sudden or nonsudden in patients with heart failure who died (Fig. 1.3) [15]. This model has been validated in several cohorts, and it has been shown to identify patients who benefitted from ICD implantation in SCD-HeFT and DANISH. As can be seen from the figure, factors that are usually associated with more advanced heart failure such as low sodium levels and high New York

Fig. 1.3 Illustration of factors that increase the relative likelihood of sudden or non-sudden death in the Seattle Proportional Risk Model

Seattle proporational risk model

Older age	Younger age
Female	Male
Higher EF	Lower EF
NYHA III or IV	NYHA I or II
Lower BMI	Higher BMI
Elevated Creatinine	Normal Creatinine
Serum Sodium <138	Serum Sodium ≥138
Diabetes Mellitus	No Diabetes Mellitus
SBP <>140 mm Hg	SBP ˜140 mm Hg
No Digoxin Use	Digoxin Use

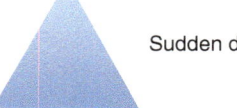

Non-sudden death   Sudden death

Heart Association Class confer a relatively higher likelihood of dying suddenly as opposed to nonsuddenly. Hence, The Seattle Proportional Risk Model indicates that ICDs are more favorable in patients with less advanced and less symptomatic heart failure.

Another way to potentially identify patients at higher risk of sudden cardiac death and hence higher likelihood of benefit from ICD implantation is by cardiac imaging. A left ventricular ejection fraction below 35% is already used as a risk marker, but it is far from perfect. Currently, most attention is paid to the possibility of using gadolinium-enhanced cardiac magnetic resonance imaging to identify localized cardiac fibrosis, which may serve as a substrate for ventricular arrhythmia. Localized fibrosis, identified by late gadolinium enhancement, is strongly correlated to the risk of overall and sudden cardiac death, and theoretically this late gadolinium enhancement might therefore serve as an indicator as to which patients should be offered an ICD [16]. However, there have been no prospective randomized studies on the effect of ICD in patients with late gadolinium enhancement, and in the subgroup of patients in the DANISH study that underwent cardiac magnetic resonance imaging, there was no sign of an increased effect of ICD in the group of patients who had late gadolinium enhancement. It therefore remains to be seen if late gadolinium enhancement on cardiac magnetic resonance imaging will improve selection of patients for ICD implantation.

An additional marker with potential for identifying risk of sudden cardiac death is bilateral ventricular dysfunction. Patients with right ventricular dysfunction in addition to left ventricular dysfunction have a much higher risk of sudden cardiac death. In the DANISH cardiovascular magnetic resonance subgroup, patients with right ventricular dysfunction lived longer with ICD implantation, whereas patients with only left-sided dysfunction did not benefit from ICD implantation [17].

Several, less common causes of nonischemic systolic heart failure are associated with a particular high risk of SCD (e.g., certain genetic cardiomyopathies) and guidelines recommend prophylactic ICD implantation for an increasing number of patients without specific trial data being available. This may be the correct strategy. However, as these patients at particular high risk of SCD have most likely been included (without knowledge of the mutation) in the trials that have convinced cardiologists of recommending ICD to patients with nonischemic systolic heart failure in general, it is likely that there are some other subsets of patients who then benefit very little from this general strategy.

Effect of ICD in Patients Who Are Candidates for Cardiac Resynchronization Therapy

Cardiac resynchronization therapy reduces morbidity and mortality for patients with left ventricular dysfunction and left bundle branch block. Patients who are candidates for cardiac resynchronization therapy often also fulfil criteria for ICD implantation. However, as the benefit of ICD implantation is related to the risk of sudden cardiac death and this risk decreases markedly with cardiac resynchronization therapy, the benefit of ICD implantation might be considerably less than in patients who do not receive concomitant cardiac resynchronization therapy. Indeed, observational data suggest this is the case [16, 18]. In addition, while the COMPANION trial did find an effect of adding a defibrillator to cardiac resynchronization therapy in patients with nonischemic heart failure, DANISH did not, and taken together, there is no statistical evidence of effect (Fig. 1.4).

Thus, there is not much evidence to support the use of defibrillators in patients with nonischemic heart failure who are candidates for cardiac resynchronization therapy. However, guidelines advocate the use of a defibrillator with cardiac resynchronization therapy, and given that the risk associated with implantation of a defibrillator electrode instead of a normal right ventricular electrode is small, it might be argued that any benefit from adding a defibrillator, however small, is risk- and cost-effective.

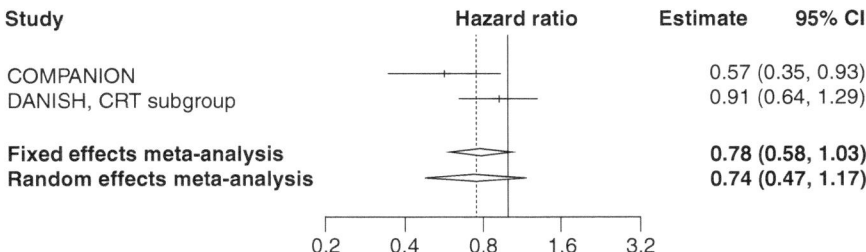

Fig. 1.4 Meta-analysis of the effect of ICD implantation in addition to cardiac resynchronization therapy on all-cause death in patients with nonsichemic cardiomyopathy. Lower hazard ratio favors ICD

Conclusion

In summary, ICD implantation for patients with nonischemic heart failure is recommended by international guidelines for secondary prevention, as well as for primary prevention in patients who are symptomatic with left ventricular ejection fraction below 35%. Further efforts to identify patients who are likely to benefit from ICD implantation are under way. In the meantime, individual patient characteristics indicating likelihood of dying suddenly should be taken into account, particularly for older patients.

References

1. The Antiarrhytmics Versus Implantable Defibrillators Investigators. A comparison of antiarrhythmic-drug therapy with implantable defibrillators in patients resuscitated from near-fatal ventricular arrhythmias. N Engl J Med. 1997;337:1576–84. https://doi.org/10.1056/NEJM199711273372202.
2. Connolly SJ, Gent M, Roberts RS, Dorian P, Roy D, Sheldon RS, Mitchell LB, Green MS, Klein GJ, O'Brien B. Canadian Implantable Defibrillator Study (CIDS). Circulation. 2000;101:1297–302. https://doi.org/10.1161/01.CIR.101.11.1297.
3. Karl-Heinz K, Riccardo C, Jürgen S, Rudolf R. Randomized comparison of antiarrhythmic drug therapy with implantable defibrillators in patients resuscitated from cardiac arrest. Circulation. 2000;102:748–54. https://doi.org/10.1161/01.CIR.102.7.748.
4. Desai AS, Fang JC, Maisel WH, Baughman KL. Implantable defibrillators for the prevention of mortality in patients with nonischemic cardiomyopathy: a meta-analysis of randomized controlled trials. JAMA. 2004;292:2874–9. https://doi.org/10.1001/jama.292.23.2874.
5. Connolly SJ, Hallstrom AP, Cappato R, Schron EB, Kuck K-H, Zipes DP, Greene HL, Boczor S, Domanski M, Follmann D, Gent M, Roberts RS. Meta-analysis of the implantable cardioverter defibrillator secondary prevention trials. Eur Heart J. 2000;21:2071–8. https://doi.org/10.1053/euhj.2000.2476.
6. Bänsch D, Antz M, Boczor S, Volkmer M, Tebbenjohanns J, Seidl K, Block M, Gietzen F, Berger J, Kuck KH. Primary prevention of sudden cardiac death in idiopathic dilated cardiomyopathy: the Cardiomyopathy Trial (CAT). Circulation. 2002;105:1453–8. https://doi.org/10.1161/01.CIR.0000012350.99718.AD.
7. Strickberger SA, Hummel JD, Bartlett TG, Frumin HI, Schuger CD, Beau SL, Bitar C, Morady F, AMIOVIRT Investigators. Amiodarone versus implantable cardioverter-defibrillator:randomized trial in patients with nonischemicdilated cardiomyopathy and asymptomaticnonsustained ventricular tachycardia – AMIOVIRT. J Am Coll Cardiol. 2003;41:1707–12. https://doi.org/10.1016/S0735-1097(03)00297-3.
8. Kadish A, Dyer A, Daubert JP, Quigg R, Estes NAM, Anderson KP, Calkins H, Hoch D, Goldberger J, Shalaby A, Sanders WE, Schaechter A, Levine JH. Prophylactic defibrillator implantation in patients with nonischemic dilated cardiomyopathy. N Engl J Med. 2004;350:2151–8. https://doi.org/10.1056/NEJMoa033088.
9. Bardy GH, Lee KL, Mark DB, Poole JE, Packer DL, Boineau R, Domanski M, Troutman C, Anderson J, Johnson G, McNulty SE, Clapp-Channing N, Davidson-Ray LD, Fraulo ES, Fishbein DP, Luceri RM, Ip JH. Amiodarone or an implantable cardioverter–defibrillator for congestive heart failure. N Engl J Med. 2005;352:225–37. https://doi.org/10.1056/NEJMoa043399.

10. Bristow MR, Saxon LA, Boehmer J, Krueger S, Kass DA, De Marco T, Carson P, DiCarlo L, DeMets D, White BG, DeVries DW, Feldman AM. Cardiac-resynchronization therapy with or without an implantable defibrillator in advanced chronic heart failure. N Engl J Med. 2004;350:2140–50. https://doi.org/10.1056/NEJMoa032423.
11. Køber L, Thune JJ, Nielsen JC, Haarbo J, Videbæk L, Korup E, Jensen G, Hildebrandt P, Steffensen FH, Bruun NE, Eiskjær H, Brandes A, Thøgersen AM, Gustafsson F, Egstrup K, Videbæk R, Hassager C, Svendsen JH, Høfsten DE, Torp-Pedersen C, Pehrson S. Defibrillator implantation in patients with nonischemic systolic heart failure. N Engl J Med. 2016;375:1221–30. https://doi.org/10.1056/NEJMoa1608029.
12. Ponikowski P, Voors AA, Anker SD, Bueno H, Cleland JGF, Coats AJS, Falk V, González-Juanatey JR, Harjola V-P, Jankowska EA, Jessup M, Linde C, Nihoyannopoulos P, Parissis JT, Pieske B, Riley JP, Rosano GMC, Ruilope LM, Ruschitzka F, Rutten FH, van der Meer P, Filippatos G, McMurray JJV, Aboyans V, Achenbach S, Agewall S, Al-Attar N, Atherton JJ, Bauersachs J, John Camm A, Carerj S, Ceconi C, Coca A, Elliott P, Erol Ç, Ezekowitz J, Fernández-Golfín C, Fitzsimons D, Guazzi M, Guenoun M, Hasenfuss G, Hindricks G, Hoes AW, Iung B, Jaarsma T, Kirchhof P, Knuuti J, Kolh P, Konstantinides S, Lainscak M, Lancellotti P, Lip GYH, Maisano F, Mueller C, Petrie MC, Piepoli MF, Priori SG, Torbicki A, Tsutsui H, van Veldhuisen DJ, Windecker S, Yancy C, Zamorano JL, Zamorano JL, Aboyans V, Achenbach S, Agewall S, Badimon L, Barón-Esquivias G, Baumgartner H, Bax JJ, Bueno H, Carerj S, Dean V, Erol Ç, Fitzsimons D, Gaemperli O, Kirchhof P, Kolh P, Lancellotti P, Lip GYH, Nihoyannopoulos P, Piepoli MF, Ponikowski P, Roffi M, Torbicki A, Vaz Carneiro A, Windecker S, Sisakian HS, Isayev E, Kurlianskaya A, Mullens W, Tokmakova M, Agathangelou P, Melenovsky V, Wiggers H, Hassanein M, Uuetoa T, Lommi J, Kostovska ES, Juillière Y, Aladashvili A, Luchner A, Chrysohoou C, Nyolczas N, Thorgeirsson G, Marc Weinstein J, Di Lenarda A, Aidargaliyeva N, Bajraktari G, Beishenkulov M, Kamzola G, Abdel-Massih T, Celutkiene J, Noppe S, Cassar A, Vataman E, Abir-Khalil S, van Pol P, Mo R, Straburzynska-Migaj E, Fonseca C, Chioncel O, Shlyakhto E, Otasevic P, Goncalvesová E, Lainscak M, Díaz Molina B, Schaufelberger M, Suter T, Yilmaz MB, Voronkov L, Davies C. 2016 ESC guidelines for the diagnosis and treatment of acute and chronic heart failure: the Task Force for the diagnosis and treatment of acute and chronic heart failure of the European Society of Cardiology (ESC) developed with the special contribution of the Heart Failure Association (HFA) of the ESC. Eur Heart J. 2016;37:2129–200. https://doi.org/10.1093/eurheartj/ehw128.
13. Al-Khatib SM, Stevenson WG, Ackerman MJ, Bryant WJ, Callans DJ, Curtis AB, Deal BJ, Dickfeld T, Field ME, Fonarow GC, Gillis AM, Granger CB, Hammill SC, Hlatky MA, Joglar JA, Kay GN, Matlock DD, Myerburg RJ, Page RL. 2017 AHA/ACC/HRS guideline for management of patients with ventricular arrhythmias and the prevention of sudden cardiac death: executive summary: a report of the American College of Cardiology/American Heart Association Task Force on Clinical Practice Guidelines and the Heart Rhythm Society. Heart Rhythm. 2018;15:e190–252. https://doi.org/10.1016/j.hrthm.2017.10.035.
14. Elming MB, Nielsen JC, Haarbo J, Videbæk L, Korup E, Signorovitch J, Olesen LL, Hildebrandt P, Steffensen FH, Bruun NE, Eiskjær H, Brandes A, Thøgersen AM, Gustafsson F, Egstrup K, Videbæk R, Hassager C, Svendsen JH, Høfsten DE, Torp-Pedersen C, Pehrson S, Køber L, Thune JJ. Age and outcomes of primary prevention implantable cardioverter-defibrillators in patients with nonischemic systolic heart failure. Circulation. 2017;136:1772–80. https://doi.org/10.1161/CIRCULATIONAHA.117.028829.
15. Levy WC, Li Y, Reed SD, Zile MR, Shadman R, Dardas T, Whellan DJ, Schulman KA, Ellis SJ, Neilson M, O'Connor CM. Does the implantable cardioverter-defibrillator benefit vary with the estimated proportional risk of sudden death in heart failure patients? JACC Clin Electrophysiol. 2017;3:291–8. https://doi.org/10.1016/j.jacep.2016.09.006.
16. Barra S, Boveda S, Providência R, Sadoul N, Duehmke R, Reitan C, Borgquist R, Narayanan K, Hidden-Lucet F, Klug D, Defaye P, Gras D, Anselme F, Leclercq C, Hermida J-S, Deharo J-C, Looi K-L, Chow AW, Virdee M, Fynn S, Le Heuzey J-Y, Marijon E, Agarwal S. Adding

defibrillation therapy to cardiac resynchronization on the basis of the myocardial substrate. J Am Coll Cardiol. 2017;69:1669–78. https://doi.org/10.1016/j.jacc.2017.01.042.

17. Elming MB, Hammer-Hansen S, Voges I, Nyktari E, Raja AA, Svendsen JH, Pehrson S, Signorovitch J, Køber LV, Prasad SK, Thune JJ. Right ventricular dysfunction and the effect of defibrillator implantation in patients with nonischemic systolic heart failure. Circ Arrhythm Electrophysiol. 2019;12:e007022. https://doi.org/10.1161/CIRCEP.118.007022.

18. Marijon E, Leclercq C, Narayanan K, Boveda S, Klug D, Lacaze-Gadonneix J, Defaye P, Jacob S, Piot O, Deharo J-C, Perier M-C, Mulak G, Hermida J-S, Milliez P, Gras D, Cesari O, Hidden-Lucet F, Anselme F, Chevalier P, Maury P, Sadoul N, Bordachar P, Cazeau S, Chauvin M, Empana J-P, Jouven X, Daubert J-C, Le Heuzey J-Y. Causes-of-death analysis of patients with cardiac resynchronization therapy: an analysis of the CeRtiTuDe cohort study. Eur Heart J. 2015;36:2767–76. https://doi.org/10.1093/eurheartj/ehv455.

Chapter 2
Risk Stratification Beyond Left Ventricular Ejection Fraction: Role of Cardiovascular Magnetic Resonance

Francisco Leyva

Introduction

In the United States, sudden cardiac death (SCD) affects 184,000–462,000 individuals per annum [1]. In Europe, annual incidence of SCD ranges between 50 and 100 per 100,000 population [2]. Although not all SCDs are due to ventricular tachyarrhythmias, up to 80% of out-of-hospital cardiac arrests are due to ventricular tachycardia (VT) or ventricular fibrillation (VF) [3, 4]. Whilst coronary heart disease accounts for most cases, around 20% are attributable to non-ischaemic causes or channelopathies.

Prominent amongst the purposes of risk stratification for SCD is the identification of patients who may benefit from implantable cardioverter defibrillator (ICD) therapy, the only life-saving therapy for patients at risk of SCD. In patient selection, clinical guidelines on primary prevention ICD therapy have adopted left ventricular ejection fraction (LVEF<30% or 40%) as the main criterion. Whilst randomized, controlled trials adopting a low LVEF as a risk stratifier have indeed shown a benefit from ICDs, it is well recognized that LVEF is a poor predictor of SCD in patients with or without cardiac disease. Moreover, most patients who succumb to a SCD fall outside the LVEF cut-offs recommended for primary prevention ICD implantation. In addition, most patients who actually receive an ICD do not develop ventricular arrhythmias (VAs) requiring ICD therapy [5].

Some authors have proposed that the myocardial phenotype could be a better predictor of ventricular arrhythmias (VAs) than LVEF [6]. Cardiovascular magnetic resonance (CMR) is now the gold standard for the characterization of myocardial phenotypes. By means of late gadolinium enhancement, CMR can inform on the quantity and patterns of myocardial scar. This review focuses on how CMR can

F. Leyva (✉)
Aston Medical Research Institute, Aston Medical School, Aston University, Birmingham, UK
e-mail: f.leyva@aston.ac.uk

© Springer Nature Switzerland AG 2019
J. S. Steinberg, A. E. Epstein (eds.), *Clinical Controversies in Device Therapy for Cardiac Arrhythmias*, https://doi.org/10.1007/978-3-030-22882-8_2

contribute to the arrhythmic risk stratification of patients with ischaemic (ICM) and non-ischaemic (NICM) cardiomyopathy and how it may help in selecting patients for an ICD.

What Is 'High Risk' of SCD?

There is no consensus as to what constitutes a 'high risk' of SCD in patients with ICM or NICM. There is, however, consensus in patients with hypertrophic cardio-myopathy. In the latter, an estimated 6% over 5 years, which equates to an annual risk of 1.2%, is considered high enough to recommend ICD therapy. However, the annual risk of SCD in ICM and NICM is as high as 2.6% (Fig. 2.1). On this basis, one could propose that a patient with ICM or NICM with an estimated 6% risk of SCD over 5 years should be considered for an ICD.

Definition of Cardiomyopathy

In the ACC/AHA/HRS 2006 Key Data Elements and Definitions for Electrophysiological Studies and Procedures, idiopathic cardiomyopathy is defined as 'heart failure and reduced systolic function without evidence of other cardiomy-opathies, including toxic cardiomyopathy, inflammatory myocarditis, valvular heart disease, tachyarrhythmia-induced cardiomyopathy, hypertrophic cardiomyopathy, cardiomyopathies associated with neuromuscular disorders and arrhythmogenic right ventricular cardiomyopathy'. Outside this definition, however, there will be patients who do not have clinical signs of heart failure, who may have reduced LV

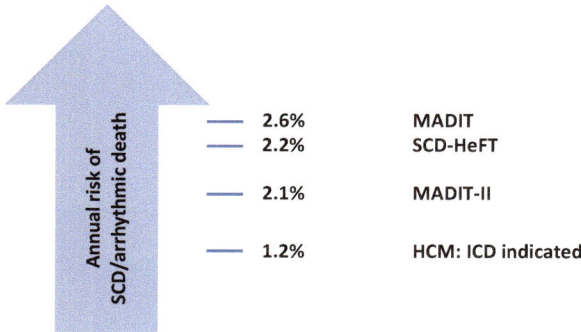

Fig. 2.1 SCD risk. Annual risk of sudden cardiac death (SCD) in the control (no ICD) arms of the Multicentre Automatic Defibrillator Implantation Trials (MADIT) and the Sudden Cardiac Death in Heart Failure Trials (SCD-HeFT) in relation to the level of risk for which an ICD is recommended for patients with hypertrophic cardiomyopathy (HCM)

function but a non-dilated LV or a myocardial scar but without LV dilation or LV dysfunction. Moreover, this definition does not specify cut-offs of LVEF or LV volumes, nor does it refer to the size or pattern of myocardial scar. To confound matters, the popular term 'NICM', referred to in device trials, is usually defined as LV dysfunction in the absence of coronary heart disease. In interpreting the findings of studies presented herein, the reader is advised to take into account variations in the definition of cardiomyopathy.

LVEF as a Risk Stratifier

LVEF is the most widely used imaging parameter in routine cardiology practice. Despite its limitations, elegantly discussed by Marwick [7], LVEF deserves credence in clinical decision-making, from the treatment for patients with MI to heart failure valvular heart disease and arrhythmias.

Few studies have explored LVEF in relation to SCD in the general population. In the Oregon Sudden Unexpected Death Study, a community-based study comprising 660,486 individuals, a retrospective assessment revealed that out of 121 SCD cases, LVEF before the SCD or aborted SCD was ≤35% in 17%, 36–54% in 22% and ≥55% in 48% [8]. The ability of LVEF to predict SCD in these patients, however, was poor (C-statistic, 0.57) (Fig. 2.2) [9]. In the Maastricht Circulatory Arrest

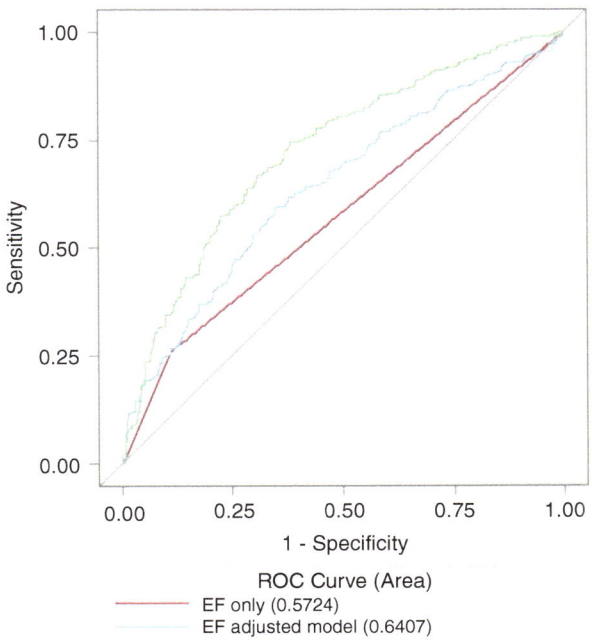

Fig. 2.2 LVEF as a predictor of SCD. Receiver operating characteristic curves for LVEF in relation to SCD. As shown, LVEF alone had poorest performance. Adjustment for age, gender, diabetes and hypertension improved performance. The adjusted model with LVEF plus ECG risk markers provided the best performance (C-statistic 0.72 vs. 0.64; $p < 0.0001$). (Reproduced with permission from Reinier et al. [9])

ROC Curve (Area)
EF only (0.5724)
EF adjusted model (0.6407)
EF adjusted model + ECG markers (0.7243)

Registry, the predictive value of LVEF was not explored, but 51% of persons suffering a cardiac arrest had an LVEF≥50% prior to the event [10].

In the context of coronary heart disease, the first evidence in support of LVEF as a high-risk prognostic marker after a MI was provided by the Multicenter Postinfarction Research Group in the 1980s [11]. In the subsequent Canadian Assessment of Myocardial Infarction (CAMI) study, the odds ratio for 1-year mortality after MI was 9.48 for patients with LVEF≤30% and 2.94 for patients with an LVEF 30–40%, compared with patients with an LVEF>50% [12]. A similar trend was observed in the Autonomic Tone and Reflexes After Myocardial Infarction (ATRAMI) study, in which cardiac mortality after MI was 7.3 higher in patients with an LVEF<35%, compared to patients with an LVEF>50% [13]. These studies showed that patients in the different LVEF categories have varying risks, but this does not equate to proof of predictive utility. This was illustrated by the Risk Estimation Following Infarction Noninvasive Evaluation (REFINE) study, in which multiple variables were considered as potential predictors of cardiac death or aborted SCD [14]. It showed that whilst patients with an LVEF≤30% had a 3.3 times higher risk of the endpoint, the receiver operating characteristic (ROC) curve was only 0.62. In the ISAR-Risk, comprising 2343 MI survivors, an LVEF≤30% emerged as a predictor of SCD at 5 years, but with a poor sensitivity (22.1%), specificity (95.4%) and positive predictive value (12.0%) [15].

In primary prevention ICD trials, there is no doubt that patients selected on the basis of LVEF derive a benefit from ICDs. In the Multicentre Automatic Defibrillator Implantation Trial II (MADIT-II) of 1232 post-MI patients with an LVEF ≤30% randomized to ICD or conventional medical therapy, mortality was lower with ICDs (14.2% vs. 19.8%) [16]. In the Sudden Cardiac Death in Heart Failure Trial (SCD-HeFT) of patients with ICM or NICM, ICD therapy was associated with a 23% reduction in mortality, compared to amiodarone [17].

Whilst a low LVEF denotes a 'high-risk' group of patients who can benefit from ICD therapy, this does not equate to LVEF being a reliable predictor of SCD. For a prognostic biomarker to be useful, it must be able to predict clinical outcomes or treatment effect, regardless of other clinical features or biomarkers. The limited specificity of LVEF in the risk stratification for SCD relates to the fact that it is a measure of pump function, rather than arrhythmic substrates. Patients with a low LVEF may therefore succumb to pump failure rather than VAs, which amounts to a competing risk. We should also consider that predicting SCD in non-ICD recipients is not the same as predicting the effectiveness of ICD therapy. In this context, the National Heart, Lung, and Blood Institute and Heart Rhythm Society report on SCD prediction and prevention has recognized the limitations of LVEF in predicting SCD [18].

Myocardial Scar and Arrhythmias: The Paradigm

Myocardial scar is a fibroblastic response to necrosis. Whilst the core of scar is electrically inert, the surrounding tissue, which consists of a borderzone of viable cardiomyocytes and fibrotic bundles [19, 20], is electrically active [21]. In the melting pot of the borderzone of scar, isthmuses with slow and fast conduction are the seat of VAs [22, 23]. Electrically, these substrates can be identified by abnormal electrograms, re-entry circuits and late potentials [24].

Myocardial Scar and Arrhythmias: Clinical Evidence

By virtue of its unparalleled ability to identify myocardial, CMR is the gold standard for the characterization of myocardial phenotypes (Fig. 2.3). Several identifiable 'imaging substrates' have been shown to relate to VAs, namely, the total amount of scar core or 'scar burden', the total amount of borderzone of scar and 'channels' within and between borderzones of scar.

Scar Core   The obvious question is whether the total amount of scar, or scar 'burden', relates to poor outcomes. In this respect, scar burden certainly relates to poor outcomes after revascularization [25–28] and pharmacologic therapy [29]. Numerous studies have also linked total scar (scar core) with SCD and VAs. In ICM, a prospective cohort study on 137 patients referred for ICD implantation showed that a scar size >5% of the LV mass adds to the prognostic value of LVEF in predicting death or appropriate ICD therapy for VAs [30] (Fig. 2.4). In a substudy of the Multicentre Automatic Defibrillator Implantation Trial II (MADIT-II), the size of myocardial perfusion defects at rest on nuclear imaging emerged as a predictor of VAs [31]. Whilst not all studies have found a link between scar burden and arrhythmic events in ICM [32] or inducibility on electrophysiological testing [33], meta-analyses do support a link [34].

The association between scar and SCD/VAs also appears to hold in NICM. Using LGE-CMR study of 65 patients with NICM undergoing ICD therapy, Wu et al. found that the endpoint of SCD or appropriate ICD shock was reached in 22% patients with CMR evidence of scar versus 8% of patients without scar [35]. In a meta-analysis of 1488 patients with NICM from nine studies, Kuruvilla et al. showed that total myocardial scar was associated with a higher risk of SCD/aborted SCD patients (6.0% versus 1.2% in patients with no scar) [36] (Fig. 2.5). In a corroborative meta-analysis, Ganesan et al. also found that presence of scar (versus absence) was associated with hazard ratio of 4.25 for SCD or ventricular arrhythmia [34]. Importantly, this association was observed in both NICM and ICM and in patients with LVEF≥35% and LVEF>35%.

Even within the positive studies showing a link between scar burden and SCD/VAs, there is no validated cut-off of myocardial scar that one could adopt as a predictor of SCD in clinical practice. Therefore, scar burden should not, by itself, be used as a predictor SCD or as indication for an ICD.

Borderzone of Scar   As discussed above, the borderzone of scar constitutes the arrhythmic substrate. Intuitively, therefore, the borderzone of scar should be a better

IMAGES	FOCUS	SEQUENCES	COMMENTS
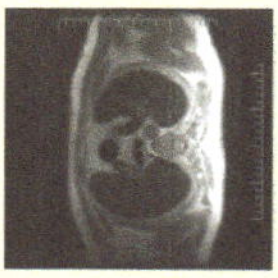	STRUCTURE	T1-weighted, contiguous slices from lung apices to diaphragm	Static 'black blood' images delineate cardiac structure
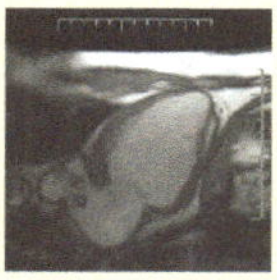	WALL MOTION	Cine steady-state-in free precession imaging (25 phases per cardiac cycle) from mitral valve place to apex	'White blood' cine images provide information on global and segmental wall motion. In post-processing, segmentation of short axis stack is used to quantify LV volumes and LVEF. Signal loss within 'white blood' indicates high velocity or turbulence
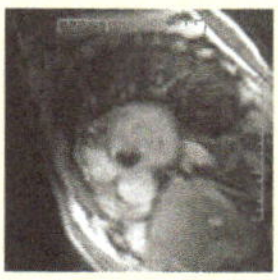	PERFUSION	Saturation-recovery imaging with gradient echo-echo planar, or steady-state-in free precession imaging 2 min after contrast administration	Perfusion defects are seen as myocardial signal loss within 2 min of gadolinium contrast administration. This can be combined with stress agents, such as adenosine.
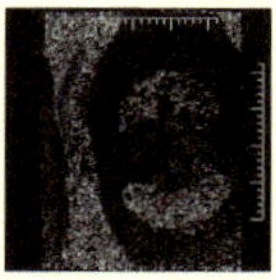	HEMODYNAMICS	Phase contrast imaging for assessment of velocity and volumes across valves.	In post-processing, velocity can be measured to assess valvular gradients.
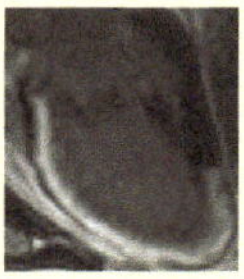	VIABILITY	Phase-sensitive inversion recovery gradient echo in short axis and long axis planes to cover entire LV, 10 min after contrast administration	In this 'white blood scan', myocardial scar appears white and viable myocardium appears 'black' after appropriate 'nulling' of viable myocardium. Signal intensity thresholds are used to define normal myocardium ($\leq$30%), scar core ($\geq$50%) and borderzoneof scar (30% to 50%).

Fig. 2.3 A CMR scan. Brief description and interpretation of a basic gadolinium enhancement CMR scan

predictor of VAs than the scar core. In an early study, Schmidt et al. found that borderzone of scar predicted inducibility for VT on electrophysiological testing, whilst neither scar burden (core) nor LVEF emerged as predictors [33]. In a study of 91 patients with a previous MI, Roes et al. found that borderzone of scar, but not scar core, predicted VAs requiring ICD therapy (Fig. 2.6) [32]. Jablonowski et al.

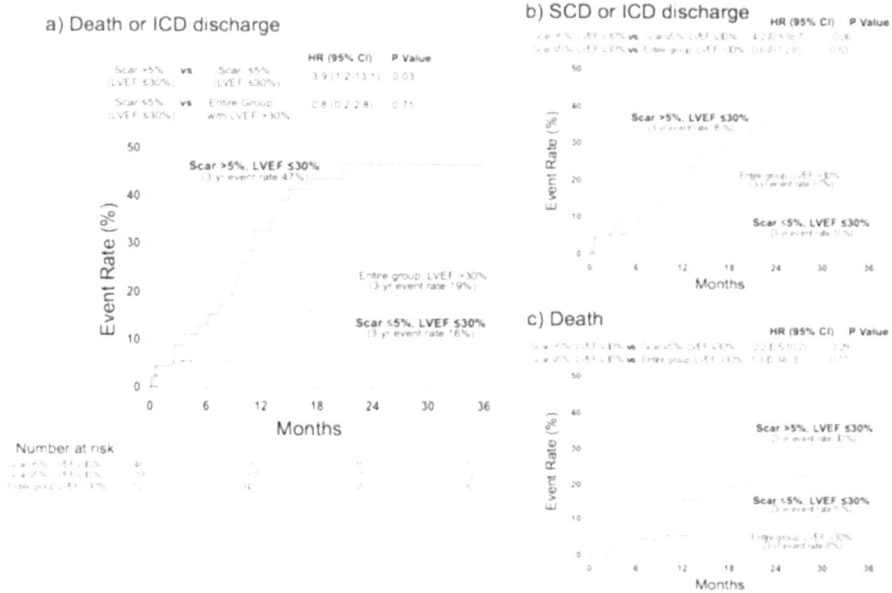

Fig. 2.4 Myocardial scar and LVEF in relation to outcomes in patients with ischaemic cardiomy-opathy. Kaplan–Meier estimates of patient outcomes according to LVEF and scar burden. As shown, patients with LVEF ≤30% and myocardial scar>5% of LV mass had a higher event rate than those with myocardial scar (≤5%) for both the primary (panel **a**) and the two secondary end-points (panels **b**, **c**). Patients with LVEF ≤30% and minimal or no scarring had similar event rate to the entire group of patients with LVEF>30%

also explored the predictive utility of different post-processing algorithms in risk stratification of patients with ICM or NICM [37]. They found that in ICM, border-zone measured by various methods consistently predicted ICD therapy (negative predictive value of 92%) in ICM. In NICM, however, only total scar and not border-zone emerged as a predictor.

Scar Patterns   Myocardial scar patterns depend on and are a marker of etiology. In coronary heart disease, ischaemia resulting from coronary artery occlusion initially leads to injury of the subendocardium. With increasing ischaemia, injury involves the mid-myocardium and ultimately the epicardium. Consequently, myocardial scar in ICM runs from the subendocardium and becomes transmural, within coronary artery territories. In contrast, myocardial injury in NICM scar is typically patchy, usually in a mid-myocardial or epicardial distribution that does not follow coronary artery territories [38].

In an early study of the relationship between scar transmurality and arrhythmo-genesis, Nazarian et al. found that scar with a transmurality of 26–75% was predic-tive of inducible ventricular tachycardia (odds ratio, 9.125; $P = 0.020$), independent of LVEF [39]. More recent studies have shown that midwall scar, which is found in

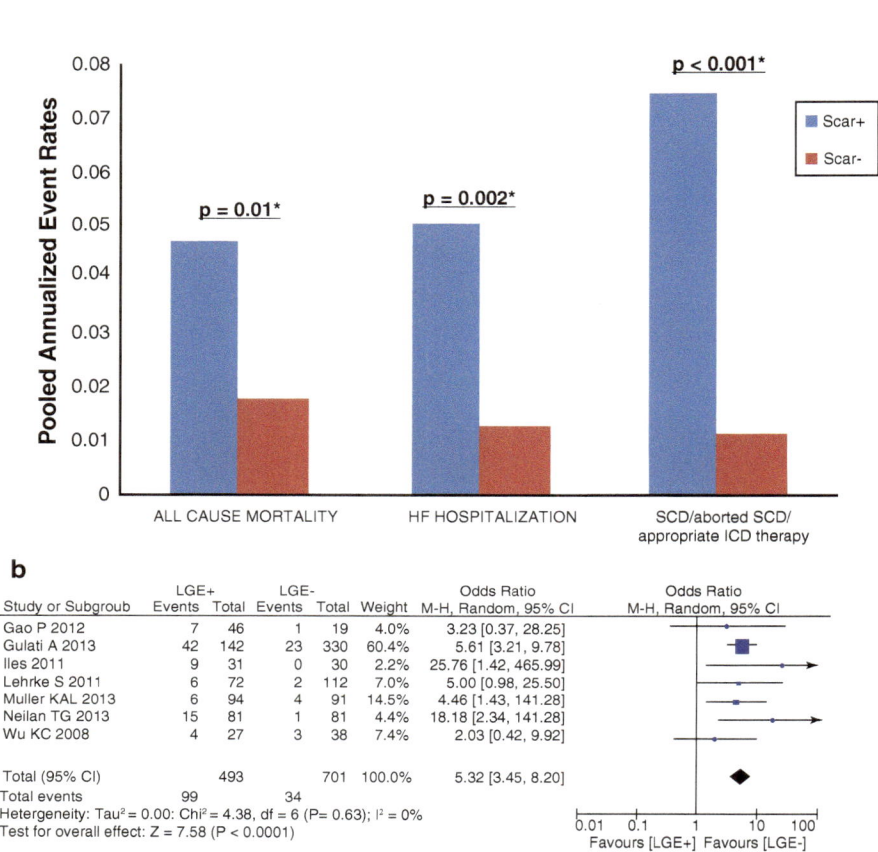

Fig. 2.5 Myocardial scar and SCD. Panel A shows weighted mean annualized event rates of cardiovascular outcomes according to the presence (+) or absence (−) of myocardial scar on late gadolinium enhancement (LGE) CMR (p values refer to scar+ and scar- groups). Panel B shows individual and pooled risk of cardiovascular outcomes for LGE CMR as well as a forest plot comparing clinical outcomes of patients with known or suspected NICM with positive LGE+ and LGE-. CI indicates confidence interval. (Adapted from Kuruvilla et al. [36])

approximately 30% of patients with idiopathic dilated cardiomyopathy, also relates to SCD and VAs. In a study of 472 patients with dilated cardiomyopathy, Gulati et al. showed that midwall scar was associated with SCD (adjusted HR, 4.61, compared to patients with no midwall scar) [40] (Fig. 2.7). In patients undergoing CRT-P, Leyva et al. found that midwall scar was associated with an 18.5-fold risk of death from cardiovascular causes [41]. In a further study from this group, cardiac resynchronization therapy with defibrillation (CRT-D) was superior to CRT pacing in patients with NICM and midwall scar, but not in patients without midwall scar (Fig. 2.8) [42].

Fig. 2.6 Borderzone of scar and outcomes. Kaplan–Meier curve analysis rate of appropriate ICD therapy when ICD recipients are stratified according to the median value of infarct borderzone (grey zone). (Reproduced with permission from Roes et al. [32])

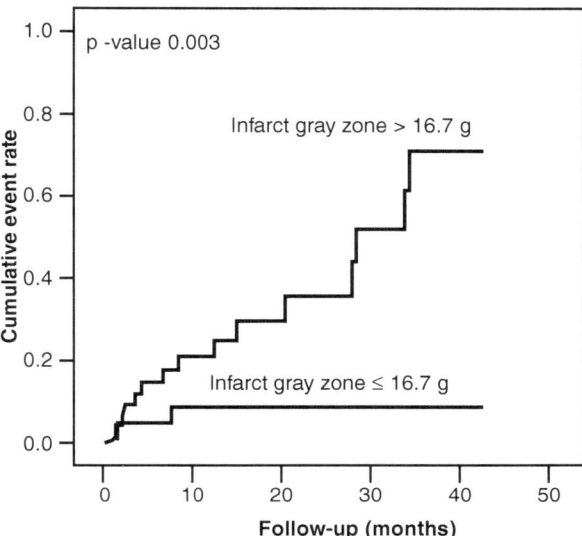

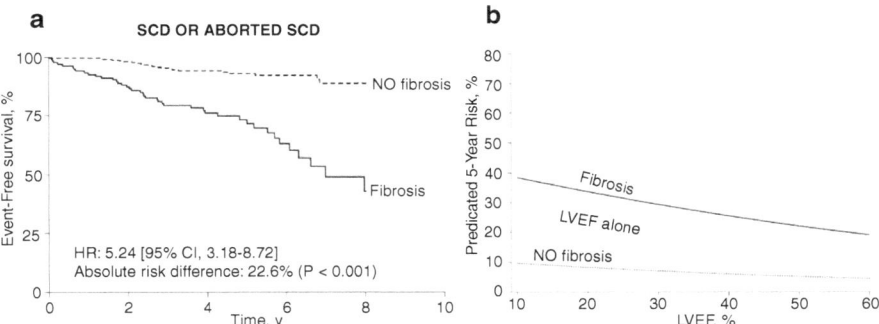

Fig. 2.7 Myocardial scar and SCD in NICM. Panel (**a**) shows Kaplan–Meier estimates of survival (left) in 472 patients with NICM patients with dilated cardiomyopathy, according to the presence or absence of myocardial scar on CMR. Panel (**b**) shows predicted 5-year risk of all-cause mortality (upper graphs) and sudden cardiac death (SCD)/aborted SCD according to LVEF. Shaded areas represent 95% confidence intervals. (Adapted with permission from Gulati, et al. [40])

Channels Continuity of borderzone of scar creates 'channels' that can potentially harbour re-entry circuits. Berruezo's group has devised a method for identifying channels using CMR (Fig. 2.9). In a study of 21 patients with MI and VT, they used a three-dimensional high-resolution 3 Tesla acquisition to explore the relationship of channels of borderzone and critical isthmuses, identified using electroanatomic mapping (CARTO). They found that CMR-defined borderzone channels identified 74% of the critical isthmus of clinical VTs and 50% of all the channels identified by electroanatomic mapping [43]. In a study of 217 patients (39.6% ischaemic), this group also showed that among patients with scar (57.6%), those with ICD therapies

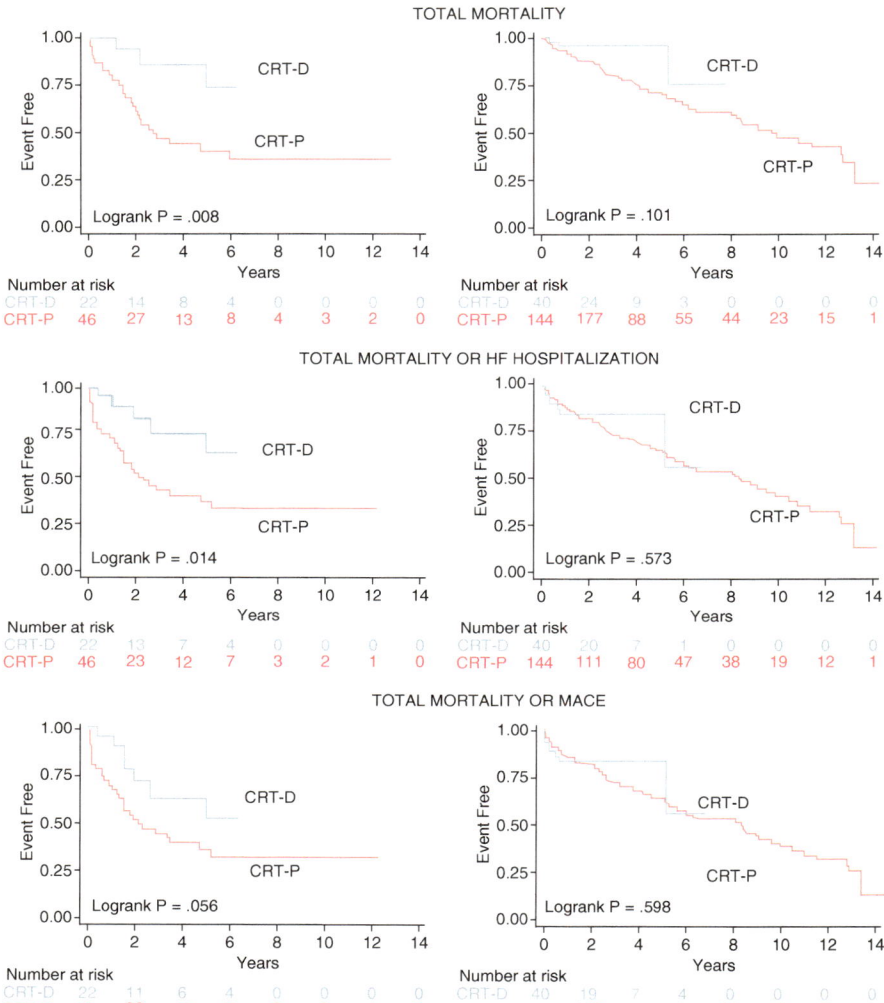

Fig. 2.8 Outcomes of CRT in patients with NICM and midwall scar. Kaplan–Meier survival curves for outcomes after CRT with (CRT-D) and without (CRT-P) defibrillation in patients with NICM, according to presence or absence of midwall scar. (Adapted with permission from Leyva et al. [42])

or SCD had the highest borderzone channel mass [44]. An algorithm based on scar mass and absence of borderzone channels identified 68.2% of patients without ICD therapy or SCD during follow-up with a 100% negative predictive value. Whilst this work provides proof of concept that CMR is able to identify the electrical substrate for VAs, it is far from providing a validated diagnostic technique that can be used in SCD risk stratification. Moreover, these findings require external validation.

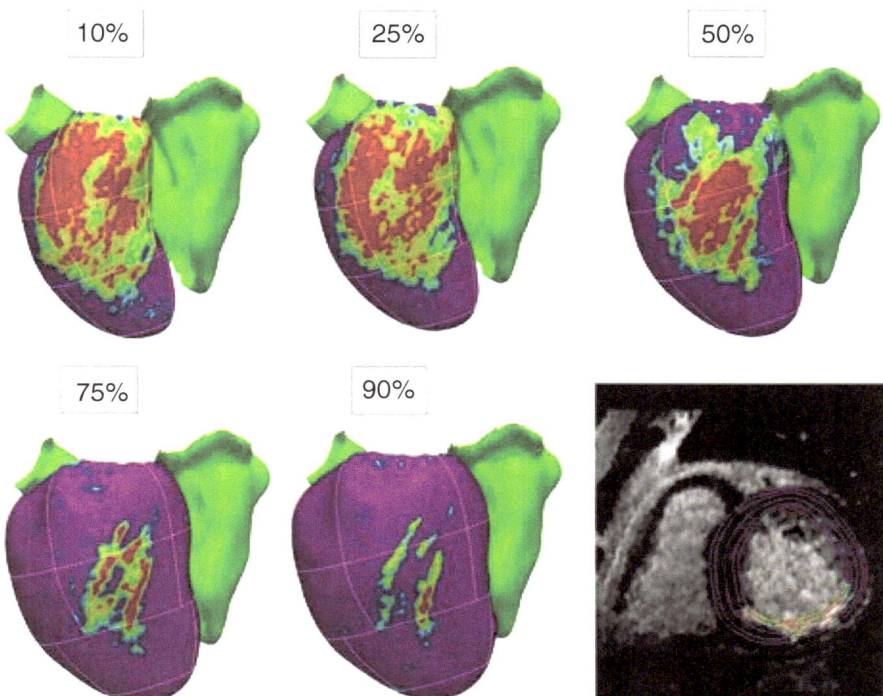

Fig. 2.9 Mapping arrhythmogenic channels with CMR. In mapping borderzone channels with CMR, concentric surface layers are created using varying cut-offs of myocardial thickness (10–90%). A three-dimensional shell is then obtained for each layer, from endocardium to epicardium. In the figure, normal myocardium is coded in purple, scar core in red and borderzone in blue, green and yellow. (Reproduced with permission from Fernandez-Armenta et al. [43])

The Future

Despite the promise of CMR in the selection of patients for ICD therapy, no randomized, controlled trials have emerged. Such trials need to test the intention-to-treat principle as to whether risk stratification on the basis of CMR is superior to echocardiographic LVEF in improving patient outcomes. The Defibrillators To Reduce Risk By Magnetic Resonance Imaging Evaluation (DETERMINE) trial, which set out to randomize 1500 patients, was discontinued because of poor recruitment [45]. The current CMR Guide Trial (NCT01918215), which includes patients with an LVEF 36–50%, may throw light on the value of CMR in selecting patients for ICDs.

Conclusions

There is no doubt that using LVEF to select patients for ICD therapy improves survival in patients at risk of SCD. Importantly, however, LVEF is ultimately a measure of pump function that is opaque to the myocardial phenotype and the arrhythmic substrate. We are currently at a juncture in deciding whether the 'imaging substrates' of VAs characterized by CMR can aid or even replace LVEF as a criterion for deciding on ICD therapy. So far, however, no scar measure or cut-off thereof has been externally validated as a predictor of SCD or benefitted from ICDs. The future of delivering the right treatment for the right patient in the field of defibrillation must surely rest on the best measures of cardiac function and myocardial phenotype that we have available. In this regard, CMR holds the most promise.

References

1. Goldberger JJ, Cain ME, Hohnloser SH, Kadish AH, Knight BP, Lauer MS, American Heart Association/American College of Cardiology Foundation/Heart Rhythm Society Scientific Statement on Noninvasive Risk Stratification Techniques for Identifying Patients at Risk for Sudden Cardiac Death, et al. A scientific statement from the American Heart Association Council on Clinical Cardiology Committee on Electrocardiography and Arrhythmias and Council on Epidemiology and Prevention. J Am Coll Cardiol. 2008;52(14):1179–99. https://doi.org/10.1016/j.jacc.2008.05.003.
2. de Vreede-Swagemakers JJ, Gorgels AP, Dubois-Arbouw WI, van Ree JW, Daemen MJ, Houben LG, et al. Out-of-hospital cardiac arrest in the 1990's: a population-based study in the Maastricht area on incidence, characteristics and survival. J Am Coll Cardiol. 1997;30(6):1500–5.
3. Bayes de Luna A, Coumel P, Leclercq JF. Ambulatory sudden cardiac death: mechanisms of production of fatal arrhythmia on the basis of data from 157 cases. Am Heart J. 1989;117(1):151–9.
4. Gang UJO, Jøns C, Jørgensen RM, Abildstrøm SZ, Haarbo J, Messier MD, et al. Heart rhythm at the time of death documented by an implantable loop recorder. EP Europace. 2010;12(2):254–60. https://doi.org/10.1093/europace/eup383.
5. Moss AJ, Greenberg H, Case RB, Zareba W, Hall WJ, Brown MW, et al. Long-term clinical course of patients after termination of ventricular tachyarrhythmia by an implanted defibrillator. Circulation. 2004;110(25):3760–5. https://doi.org/10.1161/01.cir.0000150390.04704.b7.
6. Wellens HJ, Schwartz PJ, Lindemans FW, Buxton AE, Goldberger JJ, Hohnloser SH, et al. Risk stratification for sudden cardiac death: current status and challenges for the future. Eur Heart J. 2014;35(25):1642–51. https://doi.org/10.1093/eurheartj/ehu176.
7. Marwick TH. Ejection fraction pros and cons. JACC state-of-the-art review. J Am Coll Cardiol. 2018;72(19):2360–79. https://doi.org/10.1016/j.jacc.2018.08.2162.
8. Stecker EC, Vickers C, Waltz J, Socoteanu C, John BT, Mariani R, et al. Population-based analysis of sudden cardiac death with and without left ventricular systolic dysfunction: two-year findings from the Oregon Sudden Unexpected Death Study. J Am Coll Cardiol. 2006;47(6):1161–6. https://doi.org/10.1016/j.jacc.2005.11.045.
9. Reinier K, Narayanan K, Uy-Evanado A, Teodorescu C, Chugh H, Mack WJ, et al. Electrocardiographic markers and the left ventricular ejection fraction have cumulative effects on risk of sudden cardiac death. JACC Clin Electrophysiol. 2015;1(6):542–50. https://doi.org/10.1016/j.jacep.2015.07.010.
10. Gorgels AP, Gijsbers C, de Vreede-Swagemakers J, Lousberg A, Wellens HJ. Out-of-hospital cardiac arrest–the relevance of heart failure. The Maastricht Circulatory Arrest Registry. Eur Heart J. 2003;24(13):1204–9.
11. Multicenter Postinfarction Research G. Risk stratification and survival after myocardial infarction. N Engl J Med. 1983;309(6):331–6. https://doi.org/10.1056/NEJM198308113090602.

12. Rouleau JL, Talajic M, Sussex B, Potvin L, Warnica W, Davies RF, et al. Myocardial infarction patients in the 1990s–their risk factors, stratification and survival in Canada: the Canadian Assessment of Myocardial Infarction (CAMI) study. J Am Coll Cardiol. 1996;27(5):1119–27. https://doi.org/10.1016/0735-1097(95)00599-4.

13. La Rovere MT, Bigger JT Jr, Marcus FI, Mortara A, Schwartz PJ. Baroreflex sensitivity and heart-rate variability in prediction of total cardiac mortality after myocardial infarction. ATRAMI (Autonomic Tone and Reflexes After Myocardial Infarction) Investigators. Lancet. 1998;351(9101):478–84.

14. Exner DV, Kavanagh KM, Slawnych MP, Mitchell LB, Ramadan D, Aggarwal SG, et al. Noninvasive risk assessment early after a myocardial infarction the REFINE study. J Am Coll Cardiol. 2007;50(24):2275–84. https://doi.org/10.1016/j.jacc.2007.08.042.

15. Bauer A, Barthel P, Schneider R, Ulm K, Muller A, Joeinig A, et al. Improved stratification of autonomic regulation for risk prediction in post-infarction patients with preserved left ventricular function (ISAR-risk). Eur Heart J. 2009;30(5):576–83. https://doi.org/10.1093/eurheartj/ehn540.

16. Moss AJ, Zareba W, Hall WJ, Klein H, Wilber DJ, Cannom DS, et al. Prophylactic implantation of a defibrillator in patients with myocardial infarction and reduced ejection fraction. N Engl J Med. 2002;346(12):877–83. https://doi.org/10.1056/NEJMoa013474.

17. Bardy GH, Lee KL, Mark DB, Poole JE, Packer DL, Boineau R, et al. Amiodarone or an implantable cardioverter–defibrillator for congestive heart failure. N Engl J Med. 2005;352(3):225–37. https://doi.org/10.1056/NEJMoa043399.

18. Fishman GI, Chugh SS, DiMarco JP, Albert CM, Anderson ME, Bonow RO, et al. Sudden cardiac death prediction and prevention report from a National Heart, Lung, and Blood Institute and Heart Rhythm Society workshop. Circulation. 2010;122(22):2335–48. https://doi.org/10.1161/CIRCULATIONAHA.110.976092.

19. de Leeuw N, Ruiter DJ, Balk AH, de Jonge N, Melchers WJ, Galama JM. Histopathologic findings in explanted heart tissue from patients with end-stage idiopathic dilated cardiomyopathy. Transpl Int. 2001;14(5):299–306.

20. Unverferth DV, Baker PB, Swift SE, Chaffee R, Fetters JK, Uretsky BF, et al. Extent of myocardial fibrosis and cellular hypertrophy in dilated cardiomyopathy. Am J Cardiol. 1986;57(10):816–20.

21. Nattel S, Maguy A, Le Bouter S, Yeh YH. Arrhythmogenic ion-channel remodeling in the heart: heart failure, myocardial infarction, and atrial fibrillation. Physiol Rev. 2007;87(2):425–56. https://doi.org/10.1152/physrev.00014.2006.

22. Stevenson WG, Friedman PL, Sager PT, Saxon LA, Kocovic D, Harada T, et al. Exploring postinfarction reentrant ventricular tachycardia with entrainment mapping. J Am Coll Cardiol. 1997;29(6):1180–9. https://doi.org/10.1016/S0735-1097(97)00065-X.

23. de Baker JMT, Coronel R, Tasseron S, Wilde AAM, Opthof T, Janse MJ, et al. Ventricular tachycardia in the infarcted, Langendorff-perfused human heart: role of the arrangement of surviving cardiac fibers. J Am Coll Cardiol. 1990;15(7):1594–607. https://doi.org/10.1016/0735-1097(90)92832-M.

24. Marchlinski FE, Callans DJ, Gottlieb CD, Zado E. Linear ablation lesions for control of unmappable ventricular tachycardia in patients with ischemic and nonischemic cardiomyopathy. Circulation. 2000;101(11):1288–96.

25. Allman KC, Shaw LJ, Hachamovitch R, Udelson JE. Myocardial viability testing and impact of revascularization on prognosis in patients with coronary artery disease and left ventricular dysfunction: a meta-analysis. J Am Coll Cardiol. 2002;39:1151–8.

26. Wu E, Judd RM, Vargas JD, Klocke FJ, Bonow RO, Kin RJ. Visualisation of presence, location and transmural extent of healed Q-wave and non-Q-wave myocardial infarction. Lancet. 2001;357:21–8.

27. Kim RJ, Wu E, Rafael A, Chen E-L, Parker MA, Simonetti O, et al. The use of contrast-enhanced magnetic resonance imaging to identify reversible myocardial dysfunction. N Engl J Med. 2000;343:1445–53.

28. Bellenger NG, Yousef Z, Kajappan K, Marber MS, Pennell DJ. Infarct viability influences ventricular remodelling after late recanalisation of an occluded infarct related artery. Heart. 2005;91:478–83.
29. Bello D, Shah DJ, Farah GM, Di Luzio S, Parker MA, Johnson M, et al. Gadolinium cardiovascular magnetic resonance predicts myocardial dysfunction and remodelling in patients with heart failure undergoing beta-blocker therapy. Circulation. 2003;108:1945–53.
30. Klem I, Weinsaft JW, Bahnson TD, Hegland D, Kim HW, Hayes B, et al. Assessment of myocardial scarring improves risk stratification in patients evaluated for cardiac defibrillator implantation. J Am Coll Cardiol. 2012;60(5):408–20. https://doi.org/10.1016/j.jacc.2012.02.070.
31. Morishima I, Sone T, Tsuboi H, Mukawa H, Uesugi M, Morikawa S, et al. Risk stratification of patients with prior myocardial infarction and advanced left ventricular dysfunction by gated myocardial perfusion SPECT imaging. J Nucl Cardiol. 2008;15(5):631–7. https://doi.org/10.1016/j.nuclcard.2008.03.009.
32. Roes SD, Borleffs CJ, van der Geest RJ, Westenberg JJ, Marsan NA, Kaandorp TA, et al. Infarct tissue heterogeneity assessed with contrast-enhanced MRI predicts spontaneous ventricular arrhythmia in patients with ischemic cardiomyopathy and implantable cardioverter-defibrillator. Circ Cardiovasc Imaging. 2009;2(3):183–90. https://doi.org/10.1161/circimaging.108.826529.
33. Schmidt A, Azevedo CF, Cheng A, Gupta SN, Bluemke DA, Foo TK, et al. Infarct tissue heterogeneity by magnetic resonance imaging identifies enhanced cardiac arrhythmia susceptibility in patients with left ventricular dysfunction. Circulation. 2007;115(15):2006–14. https://doi.org/10.1161/circulationaha.106.653568.
34. Ganesan AN, Gunton J, Nucifora G, McGavigan AD, Selvanayagam JB. Impact of late gadolinium enhancement on mortality, sudden death and major adverse cardiovascular events in ischemic and nonischemic cardiomyopathy: a systematic review and meta-analysis. Int J Cardiol. 2018;254:230–7. https://doi.org/10.1016/j.ijcard.2017.10.094.
35. Wu KC, Weiss RG, Thiemann DR, Kitagawa K, Schmidt A, Dalal D, et al. Late gadolinium enhancement by cardiovascular magnetic resonance heralds an adverse prognosis in nonischemic cardiomyopathy. J Am Coll Cardiol. 2008;51(25):2414–21.
36. Kuruvilla S, Adenaw N, Katwal AB, Lipinski MJ, Kramer CM, Salerno M. Late gadolinium enhancement on cardiac magnetic resonance predicts adverse cardiovascular outcomes in nonischemic cardiomyopathy: a systematic review and meta-analysis. Circ Cardiovasc Imaging. 2014;7(2):250–8. https://doi.org/10.1161/circimaging.113.001144.
37. Jablonowski R, Chaudhry U, van der Pals J, Engblom H, Arheden H, Heiberg E, et al. Cardiovascular magnetic resonance to predict appropriate implantable cardioverter defibrillator therapy in ischemic and nonischemic cardiomyopathy patients using late gadolinium enhancement border zone: comparison of four analysis methods. Circ Cardiovasc Imaging. 2017;10(9) https://doi.org/10.1161/circimaging.116.006105.
38. McCrohon JA, Moon JC, Prasad SK, McKenna WJ, Lorenz CH, Coats AJ. Differentiation of heart failure related to dilated cardiomyopathy and coronary artery disease using gadolinium-enhanced cardiovascular magnetic resonance. Circulation. 2003;108 https://doi.org/10.1161/01.cir.0000078641.19365.4c.
39. Nazarian S, Bluemke DA, Lardo AC, Zviman MM, Watkins SP, Dickfeld TL, et al. Magnetic resonance assessment of the substrate for inducible ventricular tachycardia in nonischemic cardiomyopathy. Circulation. 2005;112(18):2821–5. https://doi.org/10.1161/circulationaha.105.549659.
40. Gulati A, Jabbour A, Ismail TF, Guha K, Khwaja J, Raza S, et al. Association of fibrosis with mortality and sudden cardiac death in patients with nonischemic dilated cardiomyopathy. JAMA. 2013;309(9):896–908. https://doi.org/10.1001/jama.2013.1363.
41. Leyva F, Taylor RJ, Foley PW, Umar F, Mulligan LJ, Patel K, et al. Left ventricular midwall fibrosis as a predictor of mortality and morbidity after cardiac resynchronization therapy in patients with nonischemic cardiomyopathy. J Am Coll Cardiol. 2012;60(17):1659–67. https://doi.org/10.1016/j.jacc.2012.05.054.

42. Leyva F, Zegard A, Acquaye E, Gubran C, Taylor R, Foley PWX, et al. Outcomes of cardiac resynchronization therapy with or without defibrillation in patients with nonischemic cardiomyopathy. J Am Coll Cardiol. 2017;70(10):1216–27. https://doi.org/10.1016/j.jacc.2017.07.712.
43. Fernandez-Armenta J, Berruezo A, Andreu D, Camara O, Silva E, Serra L, et al. Three-dimensional architecture of scar and conducting channels based on high resolution ce-CMR: insights for ventricular tachycardia ablation. Circ Arrhythm Electrophysiol. 2013;6(3):528–37. https://doi.org/10.1161/circep.113.000264.
44. Acosta J, Fernandez-Armenta J, Borras R, Anguera I, Bisbal F, Marti-Almor J, et al. Scar characterization to predict life-threatening arrhythmic events and sudden cardiac death in patients with cardiac resynchronization therapy: the GAUDI-CRT study. JACC Cardiovasc Imaging. 2018;11(4):561–72. https://doi.org/10.1016/j.jcmg.2017.04.021.
45. Lee DC, Goldberger JJ. CMR for sudden cardiac death risk stratification: are we there yet? JACC Cardiovasc Imaging. 2013;6(3):345–8. https://doi.org/10.1016/j.jcmg.2012.12.006.

Chapter 3
Wearable Cardioverter-Defibrillators

Evan Adelstein, Norman Wang, and Samir Saba

Introduction

The wearable cardioverter-defibrillator (WCD) or LifeVest (ZOLL® Corporation, Pittsburgh, Pennsylvania, Fig. 3.1) is an external defibrillator that is worn by patients who are at increased risk of sudden cardiac death [1]. Through a system of electrodes contacting the patient's torso, the WCD continuously monitors the cardiac rhythm and is automatically activated if a ventricular arrhythmia is detected [2]. The WCD in its newest generation has a system of auditory and tactile alarms that notify patients if an arrhythmia is detected and a shock is imminent. Conscious patients can suspend shock delivery by actively pressing a response button designed to avoid inappropriate or unnecessary therapy delivery in the event of false-positive detection from electrode noise, benign supraventricular tachyarrhythmias, or other reasons. If an arrhythmia is detected in the absence of active suppression of shock delivery by a conscious and coherent patient, the WCD automatically releases gel from the pads in touch with the skin and delivers shocks (up to 150 J for a maximum of five shocks) to terminate the presumed lethal arrhythmia [2].

The goal of the WCD is to provide noninvasive protection of patients at high risk for sudden cardiac death (SCD) who do not have a permanent implantable cardioverter-defibrillator (ICD) [3–6]. It is often used as a bridge [5] when patients are unable to receive an ICD under various conditions, such as in the case of active systemic or localized infection or in the presence of a temporary but reversible acute illness. It is also often used when patients have an established ICD indication but cannot be implanted with a permanent defibrillator during a temporally limited

E. Adelstein
Albany Medical College, Albany, NY, USA

N. Wang · S. Saba (✉)
Heart and Vascular Institute, University of Pittsburgh Medical Center, Pittsburgh, PA, USA
e-mail: sabas@upmc.edu

© Springer Nature Switzerland AG 2019
J. S. Steinberg, A. E. Epstein (eds.), *Clinical Controversies in Device Therapy for Cardiac Arrhythmias*, https://doi.org/10.1007/978-3-030-22882-8_3

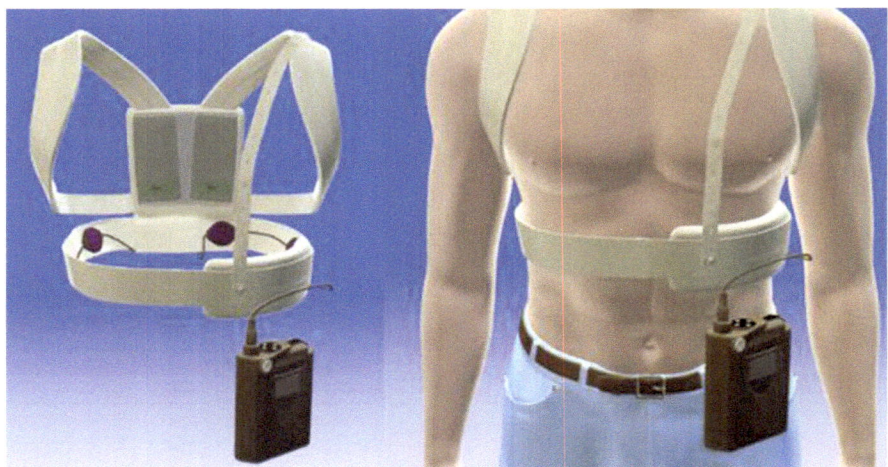

Fig. 3.1 The LifeVest (ZOLL® Corporation, Pittsburgh, Pennsylvania) is the only wearable cardioverter-defibrillator currently approved by the Food and Drug Administration of the United States

period of observation or further risk stratification such as in the first 40 days following an acute myocardial infarction or 90 days following coronary artery revascularization, or the 3–9-month period following initial diagnosis of nonischemic cardiomyopathy [3–6].

The WCD presents a significant advantage over external automatic defibrillators, as it does not require third-party intervention either for the recognition of the cardiac arrest or for physical placement of the electrode pads on the victim's chest, activation of the system, or following commands. However, what has limited its widespread acceptance is a lack of randomized clinical trials, except for the recently presented Vest Prevention of Early Sudden Death Trial (VEST) [7], which we detail in a subsequent section of this chapter, and poor patient compliance with wearing the WCD. Nevertheless, this technology has been approved by the *Food and Drug Administration* for nearly two decades and is included in the *Center for Medicare and Medicaid Services* coverage policies as well as private insurers' policies, based mainly on non-randomized, registry-type data, hinging primarily on a plausible safety profile rather than uncontroversial proof of efficacy in saving lives [8]. Despite the limited data supporting its efficacy, WCD use has expanded over the years, spurred by limitations on ICD use, concerns over the unpredictable nature of SCD, and effective corporate marketing.

Historical Landmarks in the Development of the WCD

The ZOLL® Corporation is currently the sole manufacturer of the WCD, a device actively marketed as a tool to protect against SCD but also as a cardiac monitor. The inception of the WCD dates to 1986, when a number of engineers who worked on the development of the ICD founded Lifecor, a smaller company located in Pittsburgh, Pennsylvania, that manufactured the first WCD, branded as LifeVest. Lifecor received *Food and Drug Administration* approval for the WCD in 2001 for use in adults ≥18 years of age, based on a single, non-randomized study. In 2004, ZOLL® Corporation was granted exclusive distribution rights for the LifeVest before acquiring Lifecor in 2006. In 2012, ZOLL® Corporation, which has been marketing the WCD in the United States, Europe, and Israel, entered into agreement with Asahi Kasei (Chiyoda, Japan) to promote WCD marketing in Japan [9]. Most recently in 2015, ZOLL® Corporation secured *Food and Drug Administration* approval for the use of the WCD in children between the ages of 3 and 17 years who weigh no less than 41 lbs and have a chest diameter of at least 26 in. for protection against SCD. Once again, this approval was based on a single, non-randomized study [10].

Technical Aspects of the Wearable Cardioverter-Defibrillator

The components of the LifeVest® Model WCD 3000 (Fig. 3.1) system include a garment, a monitor, an electrode belt, a holster, two lithium-ion battery packs designed for 24 h of continuous use, a battery charger, and a modem [11]. The garment has eight sizes to fit chest measurements from 66 to 142 cm (26–56 in.). While the device is designed for adults ≥18 years of age, use in pediatric patients has been described and recently approved by the *Food and Drug Administration*.

The electrode belt includes four electrocardiogram (ECG) monitoring electrodes, three therapy electrodes (or therapy pads), and a vibration box, all connected by wires. Two ECG leads available from the monitoring electrodes record side-to-side and front-to-back vectors. The therapy electrodes are configured for an apex-posterior vector. The therapy electrodes have blisters with protective coatings that contain electrolytic gel (Blue™), which is released by a signal that activates a gas-generating device sealed within the therapy electrodes. The purpose of the vibration box is to alert the patient of impending therapy. Figure 3.2a, b shows examples of successful WCD shocks delivered in response to potentially lethal ventricular arrhythmias with successful results. Figure 3.3 shows an inappropriate WCD shock delivery due to T-wave oversensing. Other causes of inappropriate WCD shocks include electrode noise, detection of supraventricular arrhythmias, or a combination of these etiologies.

ECG analysis of QRS complexes is performed using a proprietary arrhythmia detection algorithm (TruVector™) [12]. A fast Fourier transform algorithm determines the heart rate based on the strongest frequency component from independent assessments of the two ECG vectors. If the heart rate is above the tachyarrhythmia threshold, morphology analysis compares the current QRS complex to a QRS complete template previously obtained during sinus rhythm at the time of device setup. If the morphology analysis fails to match, the arrhythmia is deemed treatable. If morphology analysis is a match, therapy is not delivered, and monitoring continues. If the signal for morphology analysis is unreliable, the algorithm proceeds to heart rate, stability, and onset rhythm discrimination criteria.

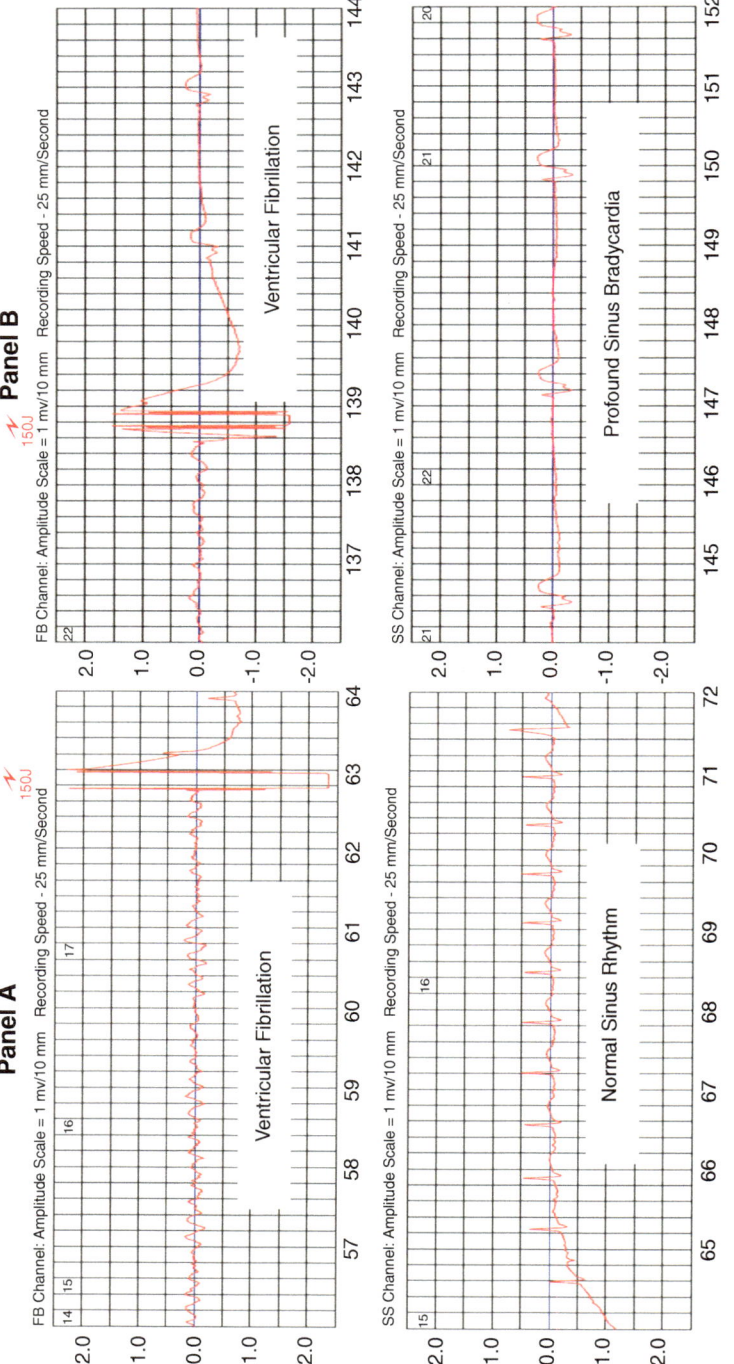

Fig. 3.2 Appropriate WCD therapies delivered in response to ventricular fibrillation in two patients. The return rhythm is normal sinus rhythm in one patient (panel **a**) and profound sinus bradycardia in the other patient (panel **b**)

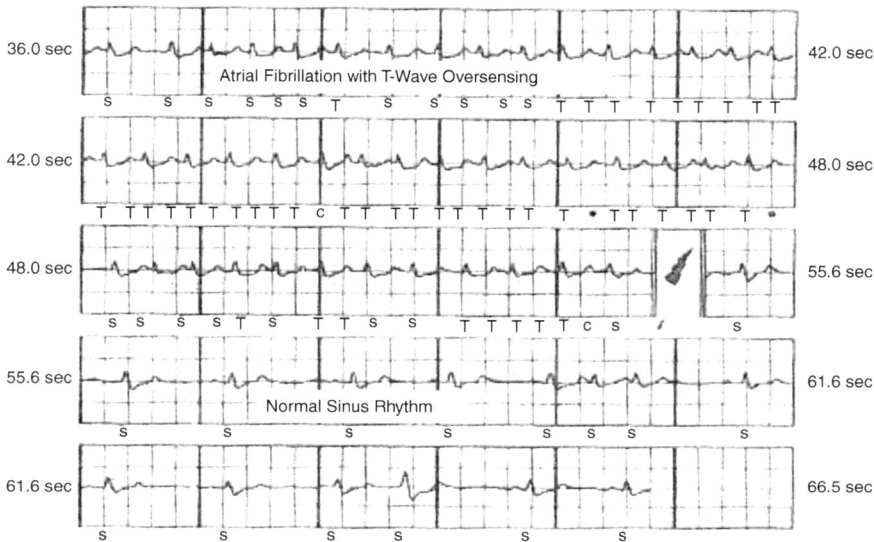

Fig. 3.3 Inappropriate WCD therapies delivered in response to atrial fibrillation with T-wave oversensing secondary to low-amplitude QRS complexes. The return rhythm after WCD shock is normal sinus rhythm with no further T-wave oversensing

The device determines the presence of a treatable arrhythmia in approximately 5–6 s, at which point the vibration alert is activated. Siren alerts then begin, and an audible verbal alert is delivered: "press response buttons to delay treatment." If the response button is not pressed, the electrolytic gel is released, and a second audible verbal alert is delivered: "bystanders, do not interfere." Finally, a shock is delivered.

Therapies may be programmed with one or two zones. The ventricular fibrillation and ventricular tachycardia zones may be set from 120 to 250 bpm. The VF zone has a default of 200 bpm and a response time of 25 s (programmable up to 55 s). The VT zone has a default of 150 bpm and a response time of 60 s (programmable up to 180 s). Delivered shocks use a biphasic, truncated exponential wave form. Up to five shocks can be delivered during an arrhythmic episode. The energy delivered is between 75 J and 150 J (±5%), programmable in 25 J increments, at 20 °C, when discharged into a 50 Ω resistive load. The software will attempt to synchronize shocks within 60 ms of the R-wave. If this cannot be achieved within 3 s, an unsynchronized shock is delivered.

The WCD function can be affected by other implantable pacing devices. Two main pacemaker interactions have been described [11]. First, if a pacemaker stimulus artifact continues during a ventricular arrhythmia, the detection algorithm may misrecognize the stimulus artifact as the QRS complex. This may result in failure to detect and treat a life-threatening arrhythmia. For this reason, the WCD is not recommended when the pacemaker stimulus artifact is greater than 0.5 mV in any ECG lead. Second, if the baseline morphology template is acquired during a ventricular paced rhythm, a native QRS complex may be interpreted as a failure to match if the heart rate exceeds the tachyarrhythmia threshold. Therefore, for those with a paced QRS complex during acquisition of the baseline morphology template, the manufacturer recommends setting the tachyarrhythmia threshold at 200 bpm.

Information from the LifeVest® can be downloaded to the LifeVest® Network for review of events [13]. High-, medium-, and low-level alerts are customizable. Notifications are triggered only for high-level alerts. Data on wear time is available and include days worn, total wear time, and average daily wear time. Newly diagnosed atrial fibrillation detected through manually recorded events has been reported [14]. Atrial fibrillation detection may have additional utility to optimize care in those with concurrently diagnosed new rapid atrial fibrillation and new reduced ejection fraction [15].

Issues with compliance with the WCD have been noted due to patient discomfort. In a national registry of over 3500 patients, 14.2% of patients with recorded data stopped using the WCD. The primary reasons cited were the size and weight of the monitor [4].

Evidence and Controversies from Clinical Trials

In this section, we will summarize the published literature regarding the WCD, provide perspective on these data, and discuss how these data have been interpreted. Most published data are derived from single-center or multicenter studies using the WCD database maintained by ZOLL®. Again, somewhat uniquely among medical devices, it was approved by regulatory agencies without randomized controlled trials, and the only randomized WCD trial has yet to be published but was presented in 2018 at the American College of Cardiology Annual Scientific Sessions. Few studies used data independent of the ZOLL® database and did not include at least one ZOLL® employee. Nevertheless, the WCD is given a class IIb indication in the most recent American Heart Association/American College of Cardiology guidelines and is therefore considered "reasonable" in patients who meet criteria for an implantable cardioverter-defibrillator (ICD) except for time restrictions [16].

The *rationale* for the WCD and thus research detailing its use is based on concerns about short-term risk of sudden cardiac death (SCD) among patients with features known to be associated with increased SCD risk in long-term studies. The lack of data, or in some populations, the publication of negative trials, has provided a niche for which the WCD allows protection against SCD without commitment to a permanent implanted device. The so-called mandatory wait period dictated by payors in patients with newly diagnosed nonischemic cardiomyopathy (i.e., within 3 months), recent (i.e., within 40 days) myocardial infarction (MI), and recent coronary revascularization (i.e., within 90 days) with left ventricular dysfunction is the most common reason for using the WCD. Some have argued for using the WCD during the oftentimes lengthy process of risk stratifying patients at potential risk of SCD [17]. Mortality after acute MI is known to be high in the early convalescent phase; in VALIANT (Valsartan in Acute Myocardial Infarction) trial, SCD was 7% within 6 months, and among those with left ventricular ejection fraction (LVEF) <30%, mortality was 2.3% in the 1st month [18]. Despite this risk, both IRIS [19] and DINAMIT [20] failed to demonstrate a survival benefit among patients with LV dysfunction in the early post-MI period.

ZOLL® Sponsored Trials

The WCD was approved based on the WEARIT/BIROAD trials [8], which were initially separate studies but were combined at the behest of the *Food and Drug Administration*. WEARIT enrolled 177 patients with New York Heart Association class III–IV heart failure and LVEF<30%, whereas BIROAD included 112 patients who had LVEF<30% at least 3 days after acute MI or coronary artery bypass graft (CABG) surgery, ventricular tachyarrhythmia within 48 h of acute MI or CABG, or resuscitated SCD/syncope within 48 h of acute MI or CABG. The study was largely a feasibility and efficacy trial; it was terminated after meeting prespecified safety and efficacy criteria. There were eight defibrillation attempts, of which six were successful, and there were additional six inappropriate shocks. Although the authors state that "most patients tolerated the device," 68 of the 289 patients (24%) stopped wearing the WCD because of discomfort or adverse reactions. WEARIT/ BIROAD used the first iteration of the WCD, which had a larger battery pack and less ergonomic garment and electrode belt than the current newest generation version.

Chung et al. published a large US registry including 3569 patients who wore the WCD a mean of 53 ± 70 days [4]. Indications for the WCD included ICD explant (23.4%), ventricular tachycardia (VT)/ventricular fibrillation (VF) before an ICD could be implanted (16.1%), genetic predisposition to SCD risk (0.4%), recent MI (12.5%), post-CABG (8.9%), nonischemic cardiomyopathy (NICM, 20%), and "unspecified cardiomyopathy" (8.1%). Eighty appropriate shocks were delivered to 59 (1.7%) patients, of whom 8 patients died despite termination of ventricular arrhythmia. Almost one-quarter of SCD were not tachyarrhythmic, consisting primarily of asystole. Only 4/546 (0.7%) of new NICM patients received a shock, of whom 1 patient died of VT/VF regardless of wearing the WCD. Limitations of this study included a lack of separation between primary and secondary prevention patients in reporting the number of patients receiving appropriate shock(s), WCD indications derived solely from the ZOLL® database, and missing clinical data. Although 16% of patients had prior sustained ventricular arrhythmias, the outcomes were reported for all patients together. There was no known indication for the WCD in 23% of patients. Also, the number of non-VT/VF SCDs was substantial, comprising 25% of total SCDs. One-fifth ($n = 12$) of 59 patients who received appropriate therapies died during that episode or before hospital discharge. Only those with an ICD explant had a relatively high risk of appropriate shocks (33 of the 59 patients who received shocks).

The ZOLL® registry was again queried in patients with recent MI (within 9 ± 9 days) and LVEF $\leq 35\%$, including 8453 patients who wore the WCD for a median 57 days [21]. There were 309 appropriate shocks in 133 patients. Of the 309 shocks, 252 terminated VT/VF, and of the 133 patient events, 121 survived the episode although 3 more patients died within 2 days. There were also 114 inappropriate shocks in 99 patients. Again, all data was from the ZOLL® database, so no medical therapy data or additional reasons why the WCD was chosen beyond LVEF were known.

The WEARIT-II Registry enrolled 2000 patients in the ZOLL® registry who were deemed high risk of SCD. It included 805 patients with ICM (40%), 927 patients with NICM (46%), and 268 patients with congenital heart disease who wore the WCD between August 2011 and February 2014 [22]. The rates of appropriate WCD therapies were 3% in ICM and congenital patients and 1% in NICM patients. Overall, there were 5 events per 100 patient-years, which was deemed a "high rate," while the inappropriate shock rate of 2 events per 100-patient years was felt to be "very low" by the authors. All appropriate shocks were successful. Nine percent of patients had a history of resuscitated SCD, and another 17% had prior syncope. Among ICM patients, 11% had resuscitated SCD and 23% had syncope. Additionally, 13% were on amiodarone, although no indications were provided. This was the first published registry to provide medical therapy data.

Independent Trials

The largest WCD experience using independent data not obtained from ZOLL® and from primary electronic medical records sources was published from the University of Pittsburgh Medical Center [23]. Over 10 years, all 639 patients with new cardiomyopathy (LVEF $\leq 35\%$) prescribed the WCD were studied, including 254 nonischemic cardiomyopathy patients and 271 ischemic cardiomyopathy patients. Median wear time was 61 days (IQR 25–102) and 22 h/day. During 56.7 patient-years of wear time, 0 nonischemic patient received an appropriate shock and 3 (1.2%) received an inappropriate shock. During 46.7 patient-years of wear time, 6 (2.2%) ischemic patients received an appropriate shock and 2 (0.7%) received an inappropriate shock. Despite appropriate WCD therapy, one patient did not survive the arrhythmic episode and one patient did not survive to be discharged from hospital. The authors concluded that WCD in patients with new ICM was reasonable but that its use in new NICM should not be routine, given the very low observed risk of VT/VF in this population.

Randomized Trials

To date, the only randomized WCD trial is the VEST, presented at the 2018 American College of Cardiology Annual Scientific Sessions [24]. This trial randomized 2302 patients within 7 days of acute MI with LVEF ≤35%, as assessed at least 8 h after presentation or percutaneous intervention or at least 48 h after CABG. One-quarter of patients had prior MI, and most were revascularized; 84% underwent percutaneous intervention, 8% received thrombolytics, and 1% had CABG. The mean LVEF was 28%, and 10% had VT/VF, presumably within the 48-h "grace period" after acute infarction. The WCD was prescribed for 90 days, during which the average wear time was 14.1 h/day and 1.4% received an appropriate shock. Inappropriate shocks occurred in 0.6% of patients. Sudden cardiac death, the primary endpoint, did not differ significantly ($p = 0.18$) between the WCD arm (1.6%) and the control arm (2.4%). There was also a statistically insignificant difference ($p = 0.14$) in non-sudden mortality between WCD patients (1.4%) vs. control patients (2.2%). Overall mortality was lower in the WCD group (3.1% vs. 4.9%, $p = 0.04$), translating into a number needed-to-treat of 56. The mechanism by which the WCD reduced overall mortality but not SCD remains unclear but possibly related to the fact that WCD wearers experience alarms and other concerns that may have increased the intensity of medical follow-up, allowing subclinical concerns to be addressed sooner.

Interpretation of the VEST trial has been controversial [25]. The study's primary endpoint, sudden cardiac death, was statistically negative. The secondary endpoint of total mortality was reduced in the WCD group, largely because of four fatal strokes in the non-WCD arm. These findings are opposite of those from DINAMIT [20] and IRIS [19], in that ICDs reduced arrhythmic and SCD in these studies but did not reduce overall mortality. The reason for these discrepant findings may be from the increased surveillance afforded by WCDs, which require more maintenance and instruction than ICDs, which are largely automated. Regardless, some have suggested that the VEST findings make prescribing the WCD reasonable in patients with recent MI and LV dysfunction.

Lack of Separation Between Primary and Secondary Prevention

Few published data describing WCD outcomes have separated patients according to primary versus secondary SCD prevention indications. It is well-established that secondary prevention patients, i.e., those with prior sustained ventricular tachyarrhythmias, have a higher future risk of SCD than primary prevention patients, i.e., those who have thus far never demonstrated sustained ventricular arrhythmias [26]. Because of this differential risk, event rates in the WCD literature may be higher than expected if secondary prevention patients are included in studies. Examples include the Chung study and WEARIT-II, in which prior sustained VT/VF was documented in 16% and 9% of patients, respectively. Only the University of Pittsburgh study specifically included patients with no prior sustained ventricular arrhythmias [23]. Because the LifeVest has been marketed to physicians for patients with primary prevention indications, we feel strongly that additional clinical trials are needed in this population, particularly in patients with NICM who have yet to be studied and who may be at a lower risk of SCD.

Current Published Guidelines and CMS Coverage

Current American College of Cardiology/American Heart Association/Heart Rhythm Society guidelines suggest a class IIb indication for the WCD [16]. This designation is the source of some controversy; as some experts have noted, this places WCD use on the same level as lenient rate control for asymptomatic atrial fibrillation [27] or using sotalol for supraventricular tachycardia in patients who do not want ablation or who are not candidates for ablation. The WCD is covered by Medicare and most commercial insurers in the United States in patients who meet accepted criteria for ICD implant but fall within the mandated "waiting period" for either NICM (i.e., 90 days from diagnosis), recent non-revascularized MI (i.e., 40 days from MI), or recent revascularization (i.e., 90 days from procedure).

Conclusion and Future Directions

The WCD is a highly effective therapy for terminating potentially lethal ventricular arrhythmias, but its impact on reducing SCD risk remains controversial. The challenges that arise when considering prescribing the WCD revolve around the low absolute risk of SCD in targeted primary prevention populations, the cost of this therapy, and the inconvenience of its use, leading to poor compliance. Potential studies of interest include randomized controlled trials in newly diagnosed nonischemic cardiomyopathies and in those who are not considered candidates for ICD implantation due to "reversible causes" of SCD [28]. From a healthcare utilization standpoint, cost-effective analyses will be important to determine the estimated cost per life saved in specific populations.

Conflicts of Interest The are no conflicts of interest for any of the authors regarding the subject matter of this chapter.

References

1. Adler A, Halkin A, Viskin S. Wearable cardioverter-defibrillators. Circulation. 2013;127:854–60.
2. http://lifevest.zoll.com/.

3. Zipes DP, Camm AJ, Borggrefe M, Buxton AE, Chaitman B, Fromer M, Gregoratos G, Klein G, Moss AJ, Myerburg RJ, Priori SG, Quinones MA, Roden DM, Silka MJ, Tracy C, Smith SC Jr, Jacobs AK, Adams CD, Antman EM, Anderson JL, Hunt SA, Halperin JL, Nishimura R, Ornato JP, Page RL, Riegel B, Blanc JJ, Budaj A, Dean V, Deckers JW, Despres C, Dickstein K, Lekakis J, McGregor K, Metra M, Morais J, Osterspey A, Tamargo JL, Zamorano JL, American College of Cardiology/American Heart Association Task Force, European Society of Cardiology Committee for Practice Guidelines, European Heart Rhythm Association, Heart Rhythm Society. ACC/AHA/ESC 2006 guidelines for management of patients with ventricular arrhythmias and the prevention of sudden cardiac death: a report of the American College of Cardiology/American Heart Association Task Force and the European Society of Cardiology Committee for Practice Guidelines (writing committee to develop guidelines for management of patients with ventricular arrhythmias and the prevention of sudden cardiac death): developed in collaboration with the European Heart Rhythm Association and the Heart Rhythm Society. Circulation. 2006;114:e385–484.
4. Chung MK, Szymkiewicz SJ, Shao M, et al. Aggregate national experience with the wearable cardioverter-defibrillator: event rates, compliance, and survival. J Am Coll Cardiol. 2010;56:194–203.
5. Klein HU, Meltendorf U, Reek S, et al. Bridging a temporary high risk of sudden arrhythmic death. Experience with the wearable cardioverter defibrillator (WCD). Pacing Clin Electrophysiol. 2010;33:353–567.
6. Lee BK, Olgin JE. Role of wearable and automatic external defibrillators in improving survival in patients at risk for sudden cardiac death. Curr Treat Options Cardiovasc Med. 2009;11:360–5.
7. http://www.acc.org/latest-in-cardiology/clinical-trials/2018/03/09/08/06/vest.
8. Feldman AM, Klein H, Tchou P, Murali S, Hall WJ, Mancini D, Boehmer J, Harvey M, Heilman MS, Szymkiewicz SJ, Moss AJ, WEARIT investigators and coordinators, BIROAD Investigators and Coordinators. Use of a wearable defibrillator in terminating tachyarrhythmias in patients at high risk for sudden death: results of the WEARIT/BIROAD. Pacing Clin Electrophysiol. 2004;27:4–9.
9. https://en.wikipedia.org/wiki/Wearable_cardioverter_defibrillator.
10. Collins KK, Silva JN, Rhee EK, Schaffer MS. Use of a wearable automated defibrillator in children compared to young adults. Pacing Clin Electrophysiol. 2010;33:1119–24.
11. https://www.accessdata.fda.gov/cdrh_docs/pdf/P010030S056d.pdf.
12. https://lifevest.mymarketingbench.com/images/1/21-90020000/20C0010.pdf.
13. http://lifevest.zoll.com/medical-professionals/lifevest-network/.
14. https://lifevest.zoll.com/sites/default/files/LifeVestNetworkCaseAFib.pdf.
15. Rodriguez Y, Althouse AD, Adelstein EC, et al. Characteristics and outcomes of concurrently diagnosed new rapid atrial fibrillation or flutter and new reduced ejection fraction. Pacing Clin Electrophysiol. 2016;39:1394–403.
16. Al-Khatib SM, Stevenson WG, Ackerman MJ, et al. AHA/ACC/HRS guideline for management of patients with ventricular arrhythmias and the prevention of sudden cardiac death: executive summary: a report of the American College of Cardiology/American Heart Association Task Force on Clinical Practice Guidelines and the Heart Rhythm Society. J Am Coll Cardiol 2018;72:1677–749.
17. Klein HU, Goldenberg I, Moss AJ. Risk stratification for implantable cardioverter defibrillator therapy: the role of the wearable cardioverter-defibrillator. Eur Heart J. 2013;34:2230–42.
18. Solomon SD, Zelenkofske S, McMurray JJ, et al. Sudden death in patients with myocardial infarction and left ventricular dysfunction, heart failure, or both. N Engl J Med. 2005;352:2581–8.
19. Steinbeck G, Andresen D, Seidl K, et al. Defibrillator implantation early after myocardial infarction. N Engl J Med. 2009;361:1427–36.
20. Hohnloser SH, Kuck KH, Dorian P, et al. Prophylactic use of an implantable cardioverter-defibrillator after acute myocardial infarction. N Engl J Med. 2004;351:2481–8.

21. Epstein AE, Abraham WT, Bianco NR, et al. Wearable cardioverter-defibrillator use in patients perceived to be at high risk early post-myocardial infarction. J Am Coll Cardiol. 2013;62:2000–7.
22. Kutyifa V, Moss AJ, Klein H, et al. Use of the wearable cardioverter defibrillator in high-risk cardiac patients: data from the Prospective Registry of Patients Using the Wearable Cardioverter Defibrillator (WEARIT-II Registry). Circulation. 2015;132:1613–9.
23. Singh M, Wang NC, Jain S, Voigt AH, Saba S, Adelstein EC. Utility of the wearable cardioverter-defibrillator in patients with newly diagnosed cardiomyopathy: a decade-long single-center experience. J Am Coll Cardiol. 2015;66:2607–13.
24. Vest Prevention of Early Sudden Death Trial and VEST Registry (VEST). ClinicalTrials.gov. https://clinicaltrials.gov/ct2/show/NCT01446965.
25. Allen LA, Adler ED, Bayes-Genis A, et al. When the VEST does not fit: representations of trial results deviating from rigorous data interpretation. Circ Heart Fail. 2018;11:e005116.
26. van Welsenes GH, van Rees JB, Borleffs CJ, et al. Long-term follow-up of primary and secondary prevention implantable cardioverter defibrillator patients. Europace. 2011;13:389–94.
27. Van Gelder IC, Groenveld HF, Crijns HJ, Tuininga YS, Tijssen JG, Alings AM, Hillege HL, Bergsma-Kadijk JA, Cornel JH, Kamp O, Tukkie R, Bosker HA, Van Veldhuisen DJ, Van den Berg MP, RACE II Investigators. Lenient versus strict rate control in patients with atrial fibrillation. N Engl J Med. 2010;362:1363–73.
28. Ladejobi A, Pasupula DK, Adhikari S, et al. Implantable defibrillator therapy in cardiac arrest survivors with a reversible cause. Circ Arrhythm Electrophysiol. 2081;11:e0055940.

Chapter 4
Cardiac Resynchronization Therapy for Heart Failure in Patients Without Left Bundle Branch Block

Valentina Kutyifa and Martin Stockburger

Abbreviations

6MWT	6-min walk test
CARE-HF	Cardiac Resynchronization-Heart Failure
COMPANION	Comparison of Medical Therapy, Pacing, and Defibrillation in Heart Failure
HF	Heart failure
LV	Left ventricular
LVEDD	Left ventricular end-diastolic dimension
LVEF	Left ventricular ejection fraction
LVESV	Left ventricular end-systolic volume
MADIT-CRT	Multicenter Automatic Defibrillator Implantation Trial–Cardiac Resynchronization Therapy
MIRACLE ICD	Multicenter InSync Randomized Clinical Evaluation Implantable Cardioverter Defibrillator trial
MIRACLE	Multicenter InSync Randomized Clinical Evaluation
MR	Mitral regurgitation
MUSTIC	Multisite Simulation in Cardiomyopathies
NYHA	New York Heart Association
PATH-CHF	Pacing Therapies in Congestive Heart Failure trial
QOL	Quality-of-life score
RAFT	Resynchronization-Defibrillation for Ambulatory Heart Failure Trial
REVERSE	Resynchronization Reverses Remodeling in Systolic Left Ventricular Dysfunction
VO2	Volume of oxygen

V. Kutyifa (✉)
Clinical Cardiovascular Research Center, Cardiology Division, University of Rochester Medical Center, Rochester, NY, USA
e-mail: Valentina.Kutyifa@heart.rochester.edu

M. Stockburger
Havelland Kliniken, Academic Teaching Hospital of Charité – Universitaetsmedizin Berlin, Nauen, Germany

© Springer Nature Switzerland AG 2019
J. S. Steinberg, A. E. Epstein (eds.), *Clinical Controversies in Device Therapy for Cardiac Arrhythmias*, https://doi.org/10.1007/978-3-030-22882-8_4

Cardiac Resynchronization Therapy

Heart failure is a global epidemic associated with high morbidity and mortality. According to recent estimates, the prevalence of HF is over 5.8 million in the USA and more than 23 million worldwide with an expected increase over time [1]. The 5-year mortality of HF is about 50%, competing with those of many cancers. Healthcare utilization associated with the care of HF is significant and costly; inpatient and outpatient visits for HF account for more than 39 billion in the USA alone [1].

Implantation of a CRT system in HF patients provided a remarkable therapeutic alternative to reduce HF symptoms and improve outcomes in advanced HF patients [2–5]. CRT is a three-lead system that delivers electrical stimuli to the right atrium, right ventricle, and left ventricle to synchronize the dyssynchronous left ventricular (LV) activation in patients with conduction abnormalities and severely reduced LV function. It should not be forgotten that CRT has been developed initially to ail the failing heart commonly impaired by three primary components of dyssynchrony: (1) atrioventricular dyssynchrony, (2) interventricular dyssynchrony, and (3) intraventricular dyssynchrony. Implantation of CRT results in an immediate decrease of intra- and interventricular dyssynchrony, a decrease in mitral regurgitation, and an increase in LV contractility [6]. During follow-up, patients exhibit a significant reduction in LV end-diastolic volume (LVEDV) and LV end-systolic volume (LVESV), and improvement in LV ejection fraction (LVEF), a process described as LV reverse remodeling [7, 8]. LV reverse remodeling is the hallmark of CRT effectiveness, and it has been shown to be directly linked to improved clinical outcomes [9].

CRT alone or the combination of a CRT with an implantable cardioverter defibrillator (CRT-D) has been proven to reduce HF symptoms, improve functional capacity, and improve quality of life in HF patients with advanced HF symptoms (NYHA class III–IV), reduced LVEF≤35%, and a prolonged QRS duration (QRS≥120 ms) [4, 5, 10]. CRT has also been shown to significantly reduce the frequency of HF hospitalizations and improve survival [4, 5]. A meta-analysis of CRT trials in advanced HF showed an overall 29% risk reduction in all-cause mortality and a 38% risk reduction in mortality due to progressive HF [11].

The Multicenter Automatic Defibrillator Implantation Trial–Cardiac Resynchronization Therapy (MADIT-CRT), the Resynchronization-Defibrillation in Ambulatory Heart Failure Trial (RAFT), and Resynchronization Reverses Remodeling in Systolic Left Ventricular Dysfunction (REVERSE) trials have further broadened CRT indication to patients with mild HF, presenting with NYHA class I and II HF symptoms [12, 13]. Figure 4.1 shows the primary results of MADIT-CRT, demonstrating a 34% risk reduction in HF events or mortality. The subsequently published long-term follow-up of MADIT-CRT and REVERSE studies confirmed sustained benefit of CRT in mild HF patients with reduction in HF events and improved survival [14, 15].

Large, randomized controlled clinical trials on the effects of CRT or CRT-D to improve HF symptoms, functional capacity, and outcomes are listed below in

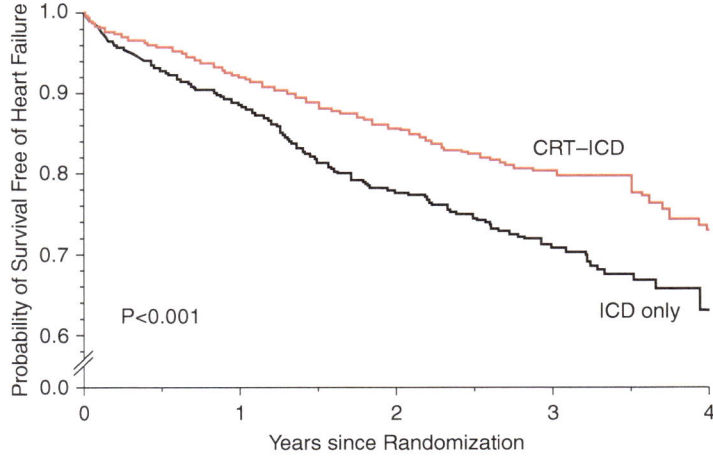

No. at Risk (Probability of Survival)

ICD only	731	621 (0.89)	379 (0.78)	173 (0.71)	43 (0.63)
CRT–ICD	1089	985 (0.92)	651 (0.86)	279 (0.80)	58 (0.73)

Fig. 4.1 Heart failure or death events in mild HF patients with CRT-D vs. ICD-only in MADIT-CRT

Table 4.1, including the respective frequencies of non-LBBB patients, when information was available. As it is evident from this table, the frequency of non-LBBB was often not reported or analyzed in the early CRT studies; these studies focused on the effects of CRT in wide QRS patients primarily presenting with LBBB. The first large randomized trials evaluating the effect of CRT on all-cause mortality, Cardiac Resynchronization-Heart Failure (CARE-HF) and Comparison of Medical Therapy, Pacing, and Defibrillation in Heart Failure (COMPANION), enrolled 6% and 29% of their patients with non-LBBB, respectively. The REVERSE study, on the other hand, enrolled 38% of patients with non-LBBB, a very high percentage, while MADIT-CRT enrolled 30% [16]. These trials also reported specific outcomes of patients with non-LBBB, allowing us to better understand differences in CRT benefit by baseline ECG morphology.

Pathophysiology of Non-LBBB

Electrical activation of the ventricles in patients with RBBB (non-LBBB) has been described by Fantoni et al. [17]. Patients with RBBB typically showed a single RV breakthrough site in the septum, as compared to LBBB with multiple breakthroughs. Following activation through the septal breakthrough site, activation then slowly spread toward the anterior region with the latest activated regions being the right

Table 4.1 Randomized controlled trials of cardiac resynchronization therapy by LBBB

Clinical trial	Patients (n)	Primary end points	Secondary end points	LVEF (%)	QRS (ms)	Non-LBBB (%)
MUSTIC-SR	58	6MWT	NYHA, QOL, peak VO2, MR, LV, hospitalizations, mortality	23 ± 7	174	13%
MUSTIC-AF	64	6MWT	NYHA, QOL, peak VO2, hospitalizations, mortality	26 ± 0	206	n.a.
PATH-CHF 2	41	6MWT, peak VO2	NHYA class, QOL, hospitalizations	21 ± 7	175	n.a.
PATH-CHF-II (Europe)	86	6MWT, peak VO2	NHYA class, QOL, hospitalizations	21 ± 7	175	n.a.
MIRACLE	453	6MWT, NHYA, QOL	Peak VO2, LVEF, LVEDD, MR, clinical response	22 ± 6	166	n.a.
MIRACLE ICD	555	6MWT, NYHA, QOL	Peak VO2, LVEF, LV volumes, MR, clinical response	24 ± 6	164	13%
COMPANION	1520	All-cause mortality or hospitalization	All-cause mortality and cardiac mortality	21	159	29%
CARE-HF	814	All-cause mortality	NYHA, QOL, LVEF, LVESV, hospitalization for heart failure	25	160	6%
REVERSE	610	HF clinical composite score	LVESVI	27 ± 7	153	38%
MADIT-CRT	1820	HF or death	LVESV, LVEDV change, multiple HF events	24 ± 5	162	30%
RAFT	1798	All-cause mortality or HF hospitalization	All-cause mortality, cardiac mortality, HF hospitalization	23 ± 5	158	20%

6MWT 6-min walk test, *CARE-HF* Cardiac Resynchronization-Heart Failure, *COMPANION* Comparison of Medical Therapy, Pacing, and Defibrillation in Heart Failure, *HF* heart failure, *LV* left ventricular, *LVEDD* left ventricular end-diastolic dimension, *LVEF* left ventricular ejection fraction, *LVESV* left ventricular end-systolic volume, *MADIT-CRT* Multicenter Automatic Defibrillator Implantation Trial–Cardiac Resynchronization Therapy, *MIRACLE* Multicenter InSync Randomized Clinical Evaluation, *MIRACLE ICD* Multicenter InSync Randomized Clinical Evaluation Implantable Cardioverter Defibrillator trial, *MR* mitral regurgitation, *MUSTIC* Multisite Simulation in Cardiomyopathies, *NYHA* New York Heart Association, *PATH-CHF* Pacing Therapies in Congestive Heart Failure trial, *QOL* quality-of-life score, *RAFT* Resynchronization-Defibrillation for Ambulatory Heart Failure Trial, *REVERSE* Resynchronization Reverses Remodeling in Systolic Left Ventricular Dysfunction, *VO2* volume of oxygen

Right Bundle Branch Block

LAO 50°

Left Bundle Branch Block

LAO 50°

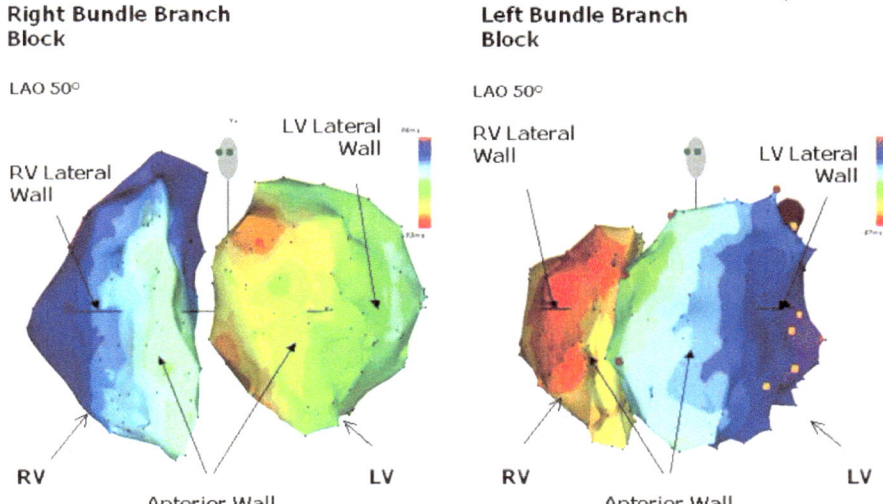

Fig. 4.2 Electrical activation of the left and right ventricle in patients with right bundle branch block and left bundle branch block

lateral wall and the outflow tract. Transseptal activation time, activation time of the RV, and total activation time were significantly longer in RBBB group compared to LBBB. In both patients with RBBB and LBBB, LV activation spread slowly, from the septal or anterior breakthrough site toward apical and lateral regions, with the posterolateral basal region being the latest activated LV area in both groups, suggesting the rationale for CRT in both patients with LBBB and RBBB (non-LBBB); however RBBB patients presented with more severe manifestation of conduction disturbances (Fig. 4.2).

Electrocardiographic Parameters to Identify Response to CRT in Non-LBBB Patients

QRS Morphology and QRS Duration

QRS duration reflects ventricular activation time. Hence QRS prolongation has great utility in informing the clinician about electrical activation delay and about regionally delayed ventricular excitation. A LBBB ECG pattern in HF patients has been related to electromechanical ventricular dyssynchrony and subsequently promotes favorable CRT effects on the failing myocardium [18], although various definitions of LBBB were associated with differences in CRT outcomes [19]. In the absence of LBBB, wide QRS may be caused by right bundle branch block (RBBB), left anterior fascicular block (LAFB), or atypical patterns of ventricular conduction delay that are frequently caused by localized myocardial scar. But in the absence of LBBB, the sole presence of ventricular conduction delay does not imply that the compromised ventricular electromechanical performance can be improved by atrio-biventricular pacing.

While the beneficial effects of CRT have been widely accepted and CRT therapy had been incorporated in all major electrophysiology guidelines worldwide [20, 21], there have been several secondary analyses reporting a suboptimal response to CRT based on the underlying ECG pattern at baseline, before CRT implantation. Specifically, patients with a left bundle branch block (LBBB) ECG pattern before device implantation have been suggested to derive a significant benefit from CRT-D, while those with non-LBBB ECG pattern were shown to have either no benefit or even a potential exposure to harm [22]. In MADIT-CRT, patients with LBBB had a significant, 53% reduction in the risk of HF or death with CRT-D versus an ICD-only (Fig. 4.3), while non-LBBB patients had a nonsignificant, 24% higher rate of HF/death with CRT-D versus an ICD-only (Fig. 4.4).

These findings have been subsequently confirmed in the REVERSE trial which found an independent relationship between QRS duration and outcomes [23]. Data from RAFT also showed a link between QRS morphology, QRS duration, and outcomes in LBBB, and similarly to our study, they did not reveal any benefit in non-LBBB patients [24]. In alignment with these findings, the National Cardiovascular Database Registry (NCDR) ICD Registry sub-study assessing CRT outcomes by QRS morphology and QRS duration confirmed that LBBB patients had better outcomes with CRT-D as compared to non-LBBB [25]. On the other hand, Cleland et al. [26] performed an individual patient-level meta-analysis combining five

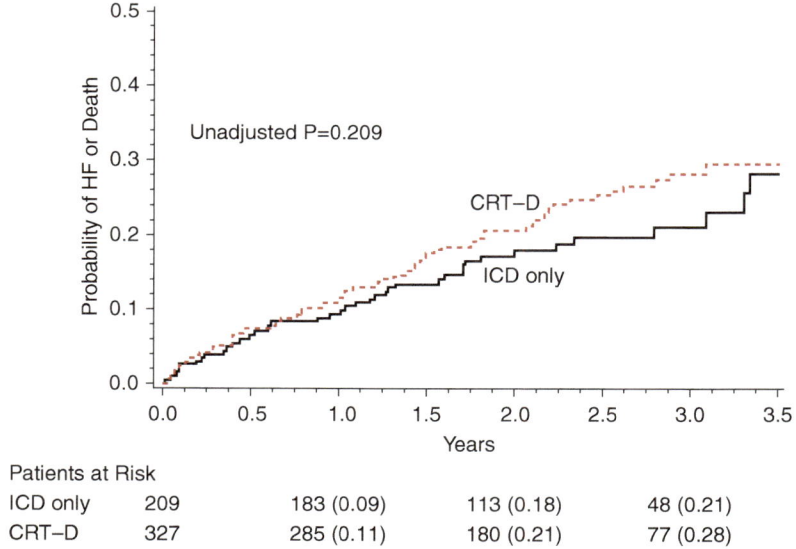

Fig. 4.3 Heart failure or death in patients with LBBB [22]

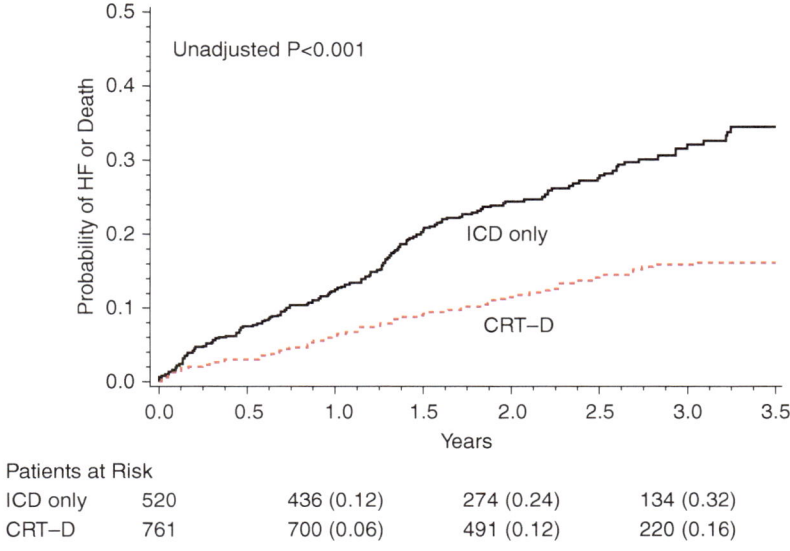

Fig. 4.4 Heart failure or death in patients with Non-LBBB [22]

randomized trials and concluded that QRS duration, but not QRS morphology, was a predictor of CRT outcomes.

In summary, QRS morphology and QRS duration appear to determine the treatment success of CRT, but prolonged QRS duration alone is questionable as a prerequisite for CRT. Accordingly, current guidelines [20] define a class I or class IIa indication for CRT in symptomatic HF patients with LBBB ≥120 ms, but non-LBBB patients do not receive a class I indication and have a class IIa indication only at a QRS duration ≥150 ms and a weaker class IIb indication at a QRS duration of 120–149 ms. HF patients with a *narrow QRS* complex <120 ms are not indicated for CRT regardless of ventricular dyssynchrony assessment, unless they require frequent ventricular pacing (>40%) to treat bradycardia [27].

QRS area assessed from the vectorcardiogram in patients with wide QRS reflects three-dimensional electrical force within the heart and has been shown to identify delayed LV lateral wall activation [28]. Therefore, QRS area has been proposed to prospectively identify CRT responders. Respective further studies to confirm this finding are under way.

Prolonged PR-Interval

A prolonged PR interval may result in atrioventricular dromopathy with compromised transmitral left ventricular filling and possible serious adverse clinical consequences [29]. A prolonged PR interval in patients without HF has been shown to be associated with an increased risk of atrial fibrillation [30], LV dysfunction, HF hospitalization, and all-cause mortality, as compared to normal PR interval [31]. This could be especially relevant in patients with established HF and conduction abnormalities, since a delay in atrioventricular conduction could further lower the cardiac output exacerbating HF symptoms [32]. Accordingly, the correction of AV coupling by CRT in HF patients with long PR interval can be hypothesized to improve the performance of the failing heart.

In line with this hypothesis, we have previously shown in a secondary analysis of MADIT-CRT that HF patients with non-LBBB ECG pattern and a prolonged PR-interval (PR ≥230 ms) derived clinical benefit from CRT-D with a 32% absolute risk reduction in HF or death at 4 years as compared to ICD (Fig. 4.4) [32]. This corresponds to a 73% relative risk reduction in HF or death and a remarkable, 81% risk reduction in all-cause mortality in this subgroup. Non-LBBB patients with a normal PR interval <230 ms derived no clinical benefit. On the contrary, patients with non-LBBB and a normal PR interval had a nonsignificantly higher risk of HF or death and more than twofold increase in the risk of death with CRT-D when compared to an ICD-only (interaction p-value<0.001) [32] (Fig. 4.5).

Such a strong bidirectional interaction with CRT-D treatment suggests that in the absence of LBBB, correction of LV dyssynchrony might not be the principal mechanism of action by CRT. It is more likely that the restoration of the physiological atrioventricular (AV) conduction by shortening the PR interval (AV delay) plays a role in the benefit from CRT-D in this cohort.

These findings were subsequently confirmed in the MADIT-CRT long-term follow-up sub-study, demonstrating sustained benefit in this cohort for up to 7 years [33]. In this follow-up study, we have also established that the benefit of CRT-D in

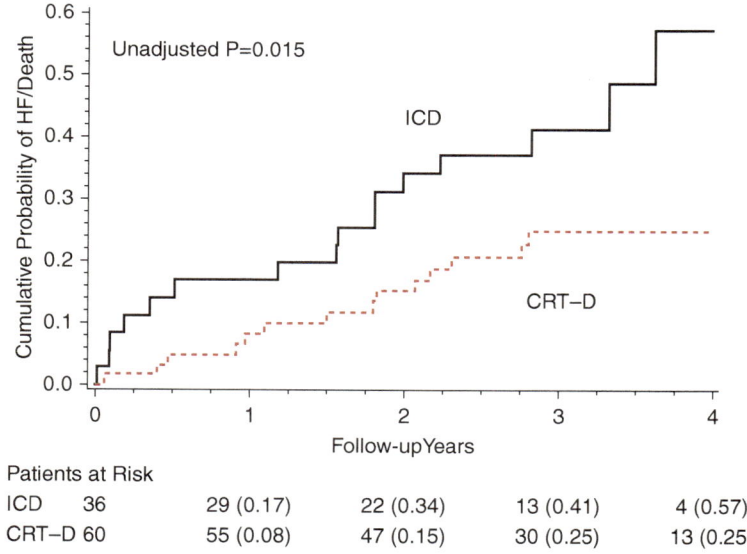

Fig. 4.5 HF or death for non-LBBB and PR ≥230 ms with CRT-D vs. ICD-only [32]

non-LBBB patients was uniformly seen for both patients with QRS <150 ms and QRS ≥150 ms. Previous studies suggested similar association with a prolonged PR interval in more advanced HF patients [34], although more recent analyses from the NCDR ICD Registry challenged these findings in a retrospective cohort study using a matched control group instead of randomization or a prospective design [35]. Therefore, these findings remain an area of controversy at this point.

The pathophysiology of a prolonged PR interval in the presence of conduction abnormalities is depicted above in Fig. 4.6. In patients with an abnormally prolonged PR interval, atrial systole (A) occurs early in diastole, and therefore, it is superimposed on the early left ventricular filling phase (E). This results in the fusion of the diastolic E and A waves, a significantly shorter effective diastolic LV filling time, and a lower cardiac output. Occurrence of an early atrial systole uncouples the mitral valve closure from LV systole resulting in diastolic presystolic mitral regurgitation, and a decreased preload and forward stroke volume, further worsening LV function. Following CRT implantation, the shortening of the PR interval to normal ranges restores the physiologic AV sequence (right panel), completely abolishes E and A fusion, and reduces or eliminates diastolic presystolic mitral regurgitation.

The underlying concept for the benefit of physiologic, AV sequential pacing in HF patients with a prolonged PR interval is well known. Previously reported case series on right ventricular (RV) DDD pacing with shorter AV delay in HF patients and low ejection fraction in the 1990s reported an improvement in HF symptoms [36]. However, in a subsequent sub-study from the DAVID trial, outcome with DDD versus VVI pacing was similarly unfavorable in HF patients with low LVEF and a prolonged PR interval (>200 ms), suggesting that dyssynchronous RV pacing in HF patients potentially outweighs the benefit of the restoration of AV synchrony [37]. We are therefore proposing that in MADIT-CRT, the presence of LV pacing (CRT) by eliminating iatrogenic dyssynchronous RV pacing while shortening the AV delay could be responsible for the above seen beneficial effects. It has also been shown

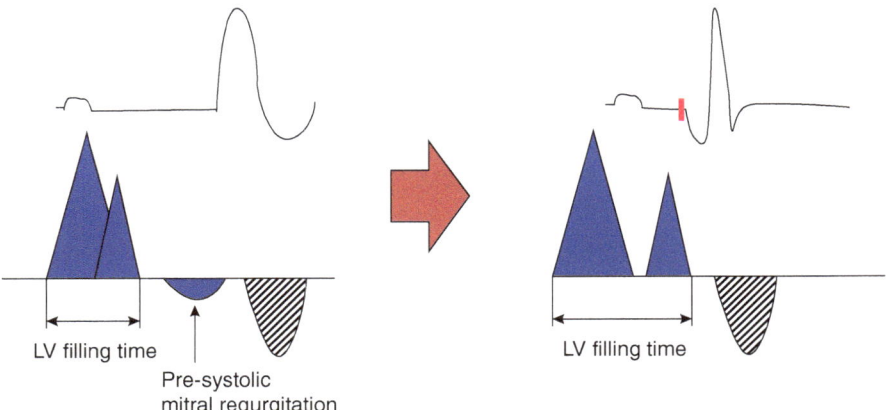

Fig. 4.6 Pathophysiology in non-LBBB with prolonged PR interval (left panel) and normalization with CRT-D and shorter AV-delay (right panel) (Kutyifa and Stockburger 2013)

that patients with first degree AV block without a pacing indication are three times more likely to develop a need for pacing during follow-up [32]. This further signifies the need for a more physiological pacing modality in this cohort, such as LV pacing. Newer techniques, such as His bundle pacing, could also be considered in this cohort, and initial studies have shown acute hemodynamic benefit in this population [38]. A larger, randomized study in patients with non-LBBB and a prolonged PR-interval applying His bundle pacing vs. no pacing is currently underway (HOPE-HF, https://clinicaltrials.gov/ct2/show/NCT02671903).

Further Electrocardiographic Parameters

A prolonged P wave duration with delayed left atrial activation may attenuate the adverse effect of a long PR on left ventricular filling. From a practical standpoint, the appraisal of the pulsed wave transmitral Doppler flow pattern may be of additional value to establish (in case of short filling and E/A fusion, Fig. 4.7a) or to disaffirm (in case of preserved E/A separation, Fig. 4.7b) a CRT pacing indication based on first-degree AV block in HF patients. Guidelines suggest a possible pacing indication in patients with a PR of at least 300 ms.

Right ventricular (RV) pacing in patients with reduced left ventricular ejection fraction has been demonstrated to adversely affect clinical outcome [39, 40]. Biventricular pacing has been demonstrated to be superior to RV pacing in AV block and impaired ventricular function [41, 42]. *Second- or third-degree AV block* with an expected ventricular pacing rate of at least 40% therefore constitutes an accepted (class IIa) indication for CRT.

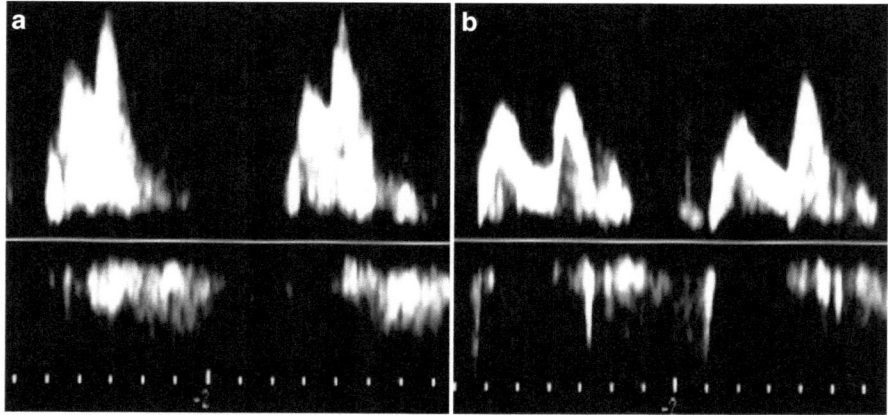

Fig. 4.7 Shortened transmitral left ventricular filling time with partial fusion of E and A waves in a patient with severe systolic heart failure, wide QRS, and long PR (panel **a**). Preserved separation of E and A waves in a patient with severe systolic heart failure, wide QRS, and normal PR interval (panel **b**)

Imaging Modalities to Identify Response to CRT in Non-LBBB Patients

It has been suggested that ventricular dyssynchrony measured during cardiac imaging could provide a mechanistically plausible and non ECG-based rationale for the application of cardiac resynchronization. Echocardiography is the most easily accessible imaging method and provides different possibly helpful variables mirroring dyssynchrony.

Two-dimensional echo (apical four-chamber view) in patients with LBBB frequently shows a typical apical left ventricular rocking movement (predominantly with counterclockwise orientation), in many patients combined with an initial septal deviation of the apex caused by early septal contraction ("septal flash"). The simple visually assessed apical rocking phenomenon has been found to predict reverse LV remodeling and a lower clinical event rate during follow-up in patients with HF and predominantly LBBB [43, 44]. The presence of apical rocking and a septal flash movement before CRT has been confirmed to predict response to CRT by a large multicenter registry [45]. However, information on the usefulness of these visual 2D echo-derived parameters in patients without LBBB is scarce.

Pulsed-wave Doppler echocardiography also adds predictive information while reliably reflecting left ventricular pre-ejection period (LVPEP) and right ventricular pre-ejection period (RVPEP) [46]. LVPEP and RVPEP are calculated as the time elapsed from QRS onset to the beginning of transaortic and transpulmonary PW Doppler flow, respectively. The interventricular mechanical delay (IVMD) is defined by the difference of LVPEP and RVPEP (Fig. 4.8).

LVPEP can be seen as a measure of global LV electromechanical performance. Baseline LVPEP prolongation of at least 140 ms and an IVMD of 40 ms or more have been shown to predict CRT response in HF patients with LBBB with high sensitivity, but limited specificity [17]. The predictive value of these parameters to predict CRT effectiveness in patients with non-LBBB HF has also been demonstrated [47]. Considering these results, Doppler echo parameters of ventricular dyssynchrony may contribute to patient-centered decision-making in the presence of HF accompanied by non-LBBB wide QRS. In addition, Doppler-derived characterization of transmitral LV inflow and atrioventricular coupling helps to anticipate possible benefit from CRT to correct the sequelae of a long PR interval.

Tissue Doppler imaging (TDI) delineates the velocity and timing of the regional myocardial wall motion in the left ventricular wall segments. Patients with LBBB usually exhibit a visually considerably dyssynchronous regional LV TDI pattern (Fig. 4.9), but numerical measures of TDI dyssynchrony were poorly reproducible and failed to identify CRT response in the Predictors of Response to CRT (PROSPECT) trial [48]. Similarly, this is true for non-LBBB.

Hence TDI-derived parameters may illustrate LV dyssynchrony, but cannot guide the decision whether to implant a CRT device in a patient with HF, but without LBBB. TDI is not able to discriminate regional myocardial contraction from passive wall motion of a scarred segment.

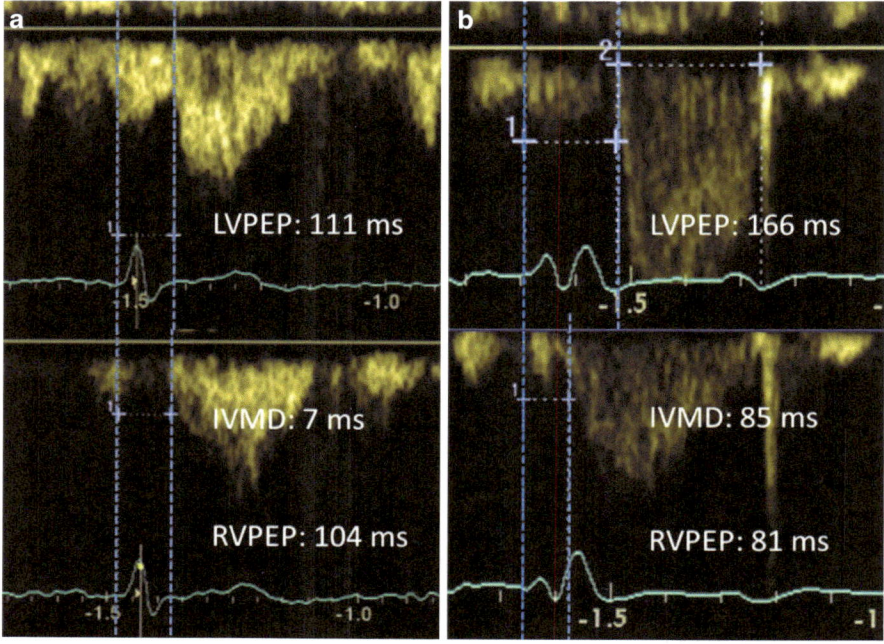

Fig. 4.8 Pulsed-wave Doppler representation of pulmonary valve and transaortic valve flow with indication of left ventricular pre-ejection period (LVPEP), right ventricular pre-ejection period (RVPEP), and interventricular mechanical delay (IVMD) from a healthy individual (panel **a**) and a patient with severe systolic heart failure and QRS prolongation (panel **b**)

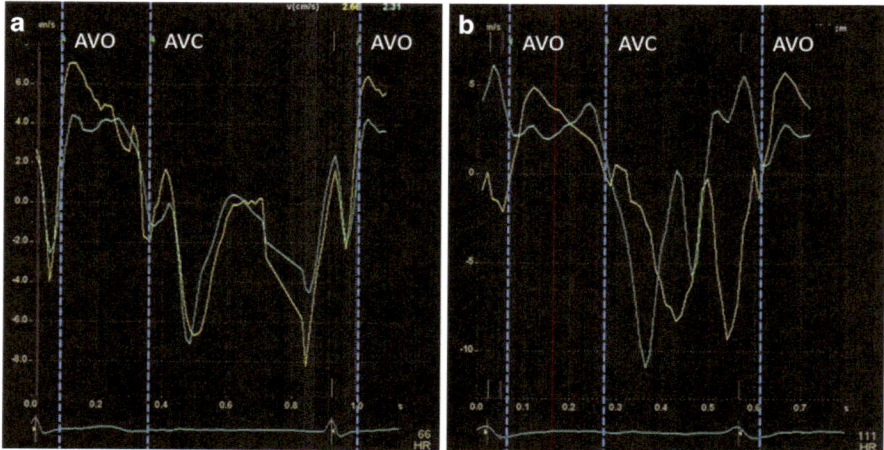

Fig. 4.9 Tissue Doppler velocity tracings with representation of basal septal and basal lateral left ventricular wall segments from a healthy individual (panel **a**) and a patient with severe systolic heart failure and QRS prolongation (panel **b**). *AVO* aortic valve opening, *AVC* aortic valve closure

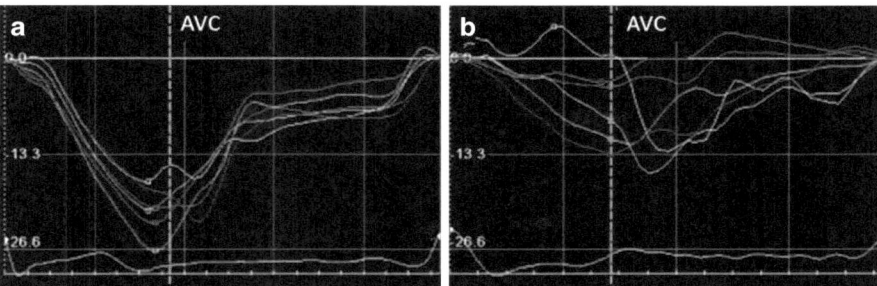

Fig. 4.10 Regional left ventricular deformation pattern assessed by two-dimensional strain imaging (speckle tracking) from a healthy individual (panel **a**) and a patient with severe systolic heart failure and QRS prolongation (panel **b**). *AVC* aortic valve closure

This methodological disadvantage is eliminated by myocardial deformation imaging modalities. Such method is two-dimensional strain echocardiography (speckle tracking). Initially, characterization of time dispersion of peak regional LV myocardial shortening (Fig. 4.10) by two-dimensional strain echocardiography (speckle tracking) showed encouraging results [49], and a derived index appeared to accurately and prospectively separate responders from nonresponders to CRT in patients with a wide QRS and heart failure. These findings were paralleled by a MADIT-CRT sub-analysis that found improving dyssynchrony and increasing global longitudinal strain to be correlated with favorable LV reverse remodeling and fewer adverse clinical events [21]. The subsequent ECHO-CRT study however did not find benefit from CRT-D versus an ICD in patients with HF, normal QRS width, and ventricular dyssynchrony derived from TDI or speckle tracking. Thus we can conclude that myocardial deformation imaging by speckle tracking can be useful to identify future CRT responders among patients with HF and a wide QRS (LBBB and non-LBBB), but probably much less so in those with normal QRS duration.

Cardiac magnetic resonance imaging (cMRI) is a promising new imaging modality that can also provide information on delayed LV ejection and abnormal apical and septal LV movement in LBBB [50] and, in addition, allows evaluating cardiac myocardial deformation [51]. However, all of these parameters can be more easily be obtained by echocardiography with sufficient reliability. The cMRI has however the most important role to localize and quantify myocardial scar, and the amount and distribution of scar may predict ventricular arrhythmias. In addition, LV pacing in scar areas should be avoided, since this could potentially contribute to ventricular arrhythmia events [52]. Therefore, cMRI can inform decision-making before CRT implantation, and it could also potentially guide LV lead placement in both patients with LBBB and non-LBBB. Image-guided CRT implantation has been shown to improve CRT outcomes in multiple trials and in meta-analysis [53]. However, it is not currently applied in standard clinical practice probably due to its time-consuming nature and its need to form multidisciplinary teams. However, further studies are warranted in this field.

Conclusions

In summary, cardiac resynchronization therapy in patients with non-LBBB has been shown to improve outcomes to a lesser degree than in patients with LBBB before CRT implantation. Additional ECG parameters, such as PR interval, QRS area, as well as imaging techniques to identify dyssynchrony, and the latest activated left ventricular segment, could be potentially relevant in this cohort to increase response rate. Alternative pacing techniques, such as His bundle pacing, are emerging to provide physiologic pacing in this high-risk population. Further studies are nevertheless warranted to better understand the pathomechanism of cardiomyopathies in patients with HF and non-LBBB, to evaluate the role of current and new treatment modalities with or without CRT, and to further improve outcomes.

Dedication The authors would like to dedicate this work to Dr. Arthur J. Moss, a true giant in cardiology, who graciously and open-mindedly allowed the authors of this book chapter to test a new hypothesis in MADIT-CRT, namely, the bidirectional relationship between PR interval and CRT-D outcomes in patients with non-LBBB. Without high-integrity leaders like Dr. Arthur J. Moss advocating for scientific curiosity freely available to anyone in the world irrespective of country, gender, sex, or age, our world would be less of many discoveries that truly advanced medicine. The legacy of Dr. Arthur J. Moss is these very discoveries and his "many sons and daughters," who will pay it forward for generations to come. We are grateful for having known him and had this opportunity.

References

1. Bui AL, Horwich TB, Fonarow GC. Epidemiology and risk profile of heart failure. Nat Rev Cardiol. 2011;8(1):30–41.
2. Epstein AE, DiMarco JP, Ellenbogen KA, Estes NA 3rd, Freedman RA, Gettes LS, et al. 2012 ACCF/AHA/HRS focused update incorporated into the ACCF/AHA/HRS 2008 guidelines for device-based therapy of cardiac rhythm abnormalities: a report of the American College of Cardiology Foundation/American Heart Association Task Force on Practice Guidelines and the Heart Rhythm Society. J Am Coll Cardiol. 2013;61(3):e6–75.
3. Brignole M, Auricchio A, Baron-Esquivias G, Bordachar P, Boriani G, Breithardt OA, et al. 2013 ESC guidelines on cardiac pacing and cardiac resynchronization therapy: the task force on cardiac pacing and resynchronization therapy of the European Society of Cardiology (ESC). Developed in collaboration with the European Heart Rhythm Association (EHRA). Eur Heart J. 2013;34(29):2281–329.
4. Cleland JG, Daubert JC, Erdmann E, Freemantle N, Gras D, Kappenberger L, et al. The effect of cardiac resynchronization on morbidity and mortality in heart failure. N Engl J Med. 2005;352(15):1539–49.
5. Bristow MR, Saxon LA, Boehmer J, Krueger S, Kass DA, De Marco T, et al. Cardiac-resynchronization therapy with or without an implantable defibrillator in advanced chronic heart failure. N Engl J Med. 2004;350(21):2140–50.
6. Breithardt OA, Sinha AM, Schwammenthal E, Bidaoui N, Markus KU, Franke A, et al. Acute effects of cardiac resynchronization therapy on functional mitral regurgitation in advanced systolic heart failure. J Am Coll Cardiol. 2003;41(5):765–70.

 7. Auricchio A, Stellbrink C, Sack S, Block M, Vogt J, Bakker P, et al. Long-term clinical effect of hemodynamically optimized cardiac resynchronization therapy in patients with heart failure and ventricular conduction delay. J Am Coll Cardiol. 2002;39(12):2026–33.
 8. Cazeau S, Leclercq C, Lavergne T, Walker S, Varma C, Linde C, et al. Effects of multisite biventricular pacing in patients with heart failure and intraventricular conduction delay. N Engl J Med. 2001;344(12):873–80.
 9. Solomon SD, Foster E, Bourgoun M, Shah A, Viloria E, Brown MW, et al. Effect of cardiac resynchronization therapy on reverse remodeling and relation to outcome: multicenter automatic defibrillator implantation trial: cardiac resynchronization therapy. Circulation. 2010;122(10):985–92.
10. Young JB, Abraham WT, Smith AL, Leon AR, Lieberman R, Wilkoff B, et al. Combined cardiac resynchronization and implantable cardioversion defibrillation in advanced chronic heart failure: the MIRACLE ICD trial. JAMA J Am Med Assoc. 2003;289(20):2685–94.
11. Rivero-Ayerza M, Theuns DA, Garcia-Garcia HM, Boersma E, Simoons M, Jordaens LJ. Effects of cardiac resynchronization therapy on overall mortality and mode of death: a meta-analysis of randomized controlled trials. Eur Heart J. 2006;27(22):2682–8.
12. Tang AS, Wells GA, Talajic M, Arnold MO, Sheldon R, Connolly S, et al. Cardiac-resynchronization therapy for mild-to-moderate heart failure. N Engl J Med. 2010;363(25):2385–95.
13. Linde C, Abraham WT, Gold MR, St John Sutton M, Ghio S, Daubert C. Randomized trial of cardiac resynchronization in mildly symptomatic heart failure patients and in asymptomatic patients with left ventricular dysfunction and previous heart failure symptoms. J Am Coll Cardiol. 2008;52(23):1834–43.
14. Goldenberg I, Kutyifa V, Moss AJ. Survival with cardiac-resynchronization therapy. N Engl J Med. 2014;371(5):477–8.
15. Linde C, Gold MR, Abraham WT, St John Sutton M, Ghio S, Cerkvenik J, et al. Long-term impact of cardiac resynchronization therapy in mild heart failure: 5-year results from the REsynchronization reVErses Remodeling in Systolic left vEntricular dysfunction (REVERSE) study. Eur Heart J. 2013;34(33):2592–9.
16. Moss AJ, Hall WJ, Cannom DS, Klein H, Brown MW, Daubert JP, et al. Cardiac-resynchronization therapy for the prevention of heart-failure events. N Engl J Med. 2009;361(14):1329–38.
17. Fantoni C, Kawabata M, Massaro R, Regoli F, Raffa S, Arora V, et al. Right and left ventricular activation sequence in patients with heart failure and right bundle branch block: a detailed analysis using three-dimensional non-fluoroscopic electroanatomic mapping system. J Cardiovasc Electrophysiol. 2005;16(2):112–9; discussion 20–1.
18. Goldenberg I, Kutyifa V, Klein HU, Cannom DS, Brown MW, Dan A, et al. Survival with cardiac-resynchronization therapy in mild heart failure. N Engl J Med. 2014;370(18):1694–701.
19. Jastrzebski M, Kukla P, Kisiel R, Fijorek K, Moskal P, Czarnecka D. Comparison of four LBBB definitions for predicting mortality in patients receiving cardiac resynchronization therapy. Ann Noninvasive Electrocardiol. 2018;23(5):e12563.
20. Tracy CM, Epstein AE, Darbar D, Dimarco JP, Dunbar SB, Estes NA 3rd, et al. ACCF/AHA/HRS focused update of the 2008 guidelines for device-based therapy of cardiac rhythm abnormalities: a report of the American College of Cardiology Foundation/American Heart Association Task Force on Practice Guidelines. Heart Rhythm. 2012;9(10):1737–53.
21. Priori SG, Blomstrom-Lundqvist C, Mazzanti A, Blom N, Borggrefe M, Camm J, et al. 2015 ESC guidelines for the management of patients with ventricular arrhythmias and the prevention of sudden cardiac death: the Task Force for the Management of Patients with Ventricular Arrhythmias and the Prevention of Sudden Cardiac Death of the European Society of Cardiology (ESC). Endorsed by: Association for European Paediatric and Congenital Cardiology (AEPC). Eur Heart J. 2015;36(41):2793–867.
22. Zareba W, Klein H, Cygankiewicz I, Hall WJ, McNitt S, Brown M, et al. Effectiveness of cardiac resynchronization therapy by QRS morphology in the Multicenter Automatic Defibrillator

Implantation Trial-Cardiac Resynchronization Therapy (MADIT-CRT). Circulation. 2011;123(10):1061–72.
23. Gold MR, Thebault C, Linde C, Abraham WT, Gerritse B, Ghio S, et al. Effect of QRS duration and morphology on cardiac resynchronization therapy outcomes in mild heart failure: results from the Resynchronization Reverses Remodeling in Systolic Left Ventricular Dysfunction (REVERSE) study. Circulation. 2012;126(7):822–9.
24. Birnie DH, Ha A, Higginson L, Sidhu K, Green M, Philippon F, et al. Impact of QRS morphology and duration on outcomes after cardiac resynchronization therapy: results from the Resynchronization-Defibrillation for Ambulatory Heart Failure Trial (RAFT). Circ Heart Fail. 2013;6(6):1190–8.
25. Peterson PN, Greiner MA, Qualls LG, Al-Khatib SM, Curtis JP, Fonarow GC, et al. QRS duration, bundle-branch block morphology, and outcomes among older patients with heart failure receiving cardiac resynchronization therapy. JAMA. 2013;310(6):617–26.
26. Cleland JG, Abraham WT, Linde C, Gold MR, Young JB, Claude Daubert J, et al. An individual patient meta-analysis of five randomized trials assessing the effects of cardiac resynchronization therapy on morbidity and mortality in patients with symptomatic heart failure. Eur Heart J. 2013;34(46):3547–56.
27. Ruschitzka F, Abraham WT, Singh JP, Bax JJ, Borer JS, Brugada J, et al. Cardiac-resynchronization therapy in heart failure with a narrow QRS complex. N Engl J Med. 2013;369(15):1395–405.
28. van Stipdonk AMW, Ter Horst I, Kloosterman M, Engels EB, Rienstra M, Crijns H, et al. QRS area is a strong determinant of outcome in cardiac resynchronization therapy. Circ Arrhythm Electrophysiol. 2018;11(12):e006497.
29. Salden F, Kutyifa V, Stockburger M, Prinzen FW, Vernooy K. Atrioventricular dromotropathy: evidence for a distinctive entity in heart failure with prolonged PR interval? Europace. 2018;20(7):1067–77.
30. Cheng S, Keyes MJ, Larson MG, McCabe EL, Newton-Cheh C, Levy D, et al. Long-term outcomes in individuals with prolonged PR interval or first-degree atrioventricular block. JAMA. 2009;301(24):2571–7.
31. Crisel RK, Farzaneh-Far R, Na B, Whooley MA. First-degree atrioventricular block is associated with heart failure and death in persons with stable coronary artery disease: data from the Heart and Soul Study. Eur Heart J. 2011;32(15):1875–80.
32. Kutyifa V, Stockburger M, Daubert JP, Holmqvist F, Olshansky B, Schuger C, et al. PR interval identifies clinical response in patients with non-left bundle branch block: a Multicenter Automatic Defibrillator Implantation Trial-Cardiac Resynchronization Therapy substudy. Circ Arrhythm Electrophysiol. 2014;7(4):645–51.
33. Stockburger M, Moss AJ, Klein HU, Zareba W, Goldenberg I, Biton Y, et al. Sustained clinical benefit of cardiac resynchronization therapy in non-LBBB patients with prolonged PR-interval: MADIT-CRT long-term follow-up. Clin Res Cardiol. 2016;105(11):944–52.
34. Olshansky B, Day JD, Sullivan RM, Yong P, Galle E, Steinberg JS. Does cardiac resynchronization therapy provide unrecognized benefit in patients with prolonged PR intervals? The impact of restoring atrioventricular synchrony: an analysis from the COMPANION trial. Heart Rhythm. 2012;9(1):34–9.
35. Friedman DJ, Bao H, Spatz ES, Curtis JP, Daubert JP, Al-Khatib SM. Association between a prolonged PR interval and outcomes of cardiac resynchronization therapy: a report from the National Cardiovascular Data Registry. Circulation. 2016;134(21):1617–28.
36. Hochleitner M, Hortnagl H, Ng CK, Gschnitzer F, Zechmann W. Usefulness of physiologic dual-chamber pacing in drug-resistant idiopathic dilated cardiomyopathy. Am J Cardiol. 1990;66(2):198–202.
37. Kutalek SP, Sharma AD, McWilliams MJ, Wilkoff BL, Leonen A, Hallstrom AP, et al. Effect of pacing for soft indications on mortality and heart failure in the dual chamber and VVI implantable defibrillator (DAVID) trial. Pacing Clin Electrophysiol (PACE). 2008;31(7):828–37.

38. Sohaib SMA, Wright I, Lim E, Moore P, Lim PB, Koawing M, et al. Atrioventricular optimized direct his bundle pacing improves acute hemodynamic function in patients with heart failure and PR interval prolongation without left bundle branch block. JACC Clin Electrophysiol. 2015;1(6):582–91.

39. Steinberg JS, Fischer A, Wang P, Schuger C, Daubert J, McNitt S, et al. The clinical implications of cumulative right ventricular pacing in the multicenter automatic defibrillator trial II. J Cardiovasc Electrophysiol. 2005;16(4):359–65.

40. Wilkoff BL, Cook JR, Epstein AE, Greene HL, Hallstrom AP, Hsia H, et al. Dual-chamber pacing or ventricular backup pacing in patients with an implantable defibrillator: the Dual Chamber and VVI Implantable Defibrillator (DAVID) trial. JAMA. 2002;288(24):3115–23.

41. Curtis AB, Worley SJ, Adamson PB, Chung ES, Niazi I, Sherfesee L, et al. Biventricular pacing for atrioventricular block and systolic dysfunction. N Engl J Med. 2013;368(17):1585–93.

42. Kindermann M, Hennen B, Jung J, Geisel J, Bohm M, Frohlig G. Biventricular versus conventional right ventricular stimulation for patients with standard pacing indication and left ventricular dysfunction: the Homburg Biventricular Pacing Evaluation (HOBIPACE). J Am Coll Cardiol. 2006;47(10):1927–37.

43. Ghani A, Delnoy PP, Ottervanger JP, Ramdat Misier AR, Smit JJ, Adiyaman A, et al. Association of apical rocking with long-term major adverse cardiac events in patients undergoing cardiac resynchronization therapy. Eur Heart J Cardiovasc Imaging. 2016;17(2):146–53.

44. Ghani A, Delnoy PP, Ottervanger JP, Misier AR, Smit JJ, Adiyaman A, et al. Apical rocking is predictive of response to cardiac resynchronization therapy. Int J Cardiovasc Imaging. 2015;31(4):717–25.

45. Beela AS, Unlu S, Duchenne J, Ciarka A, Daraban AM, Kotrc M, et al. Assessment of mechanical dyssynchrony can improve the prognostic value of guideline-based patient selection for cardiac resynchronization therapy. Eur Heart J Cardiovasc Imaging. 2019;20(1):66–74.

46. Stockburger M, Fateh-Moghadam S, Nitardy A, Celebi O, Krebs A, Habedank D, et al. Baseline Doppler parameters are useful predictors of chronic left ventricular reduction in size by cardiac resynchronization therapy. Europace. 2008;10(1):69–74.

47. Hara H, Oyenuga OA, Tanaka H, Adelstein EC, Onishi T, McNamara DM, et al. The relationship of QRS morphology and mechanical dyssynchrony to long-term outcome following cardiac resynchronization therapy. Eur Heart J. 2012;33(21):2680–91.

48. Chung ES, Leon AR, Tavazzi L, Sun JP, Nihoyannopoulos P, Merlino J, et al. Results of the predictors of response to CRT (PROSPECT) trial. Circulation. 2008;117(20):2608–16.

49. Lim P, Buakhamsri A, Popovic ZB, Greenberg NL, Patel D, Thomas JD, et al. Longitudinal strain delay index by speckle tracking imaging: a new marker of response to cardiac resynchronization therapy. Circulation. 2008;118(11):1130–7.

50. Revah G, Wu V, Huntjens PR, Piekarski E, Chyou JY, Axel L. Cardiovascular magnetic resonance features of mechanical dyssynchrony in patients with left bundle branch block. Int J Cardiovasc Imaging. 2016;32(9):1427–38.

51. Zweerink A, van Everdingen WM, Nijveldt R, Salden OAE, Meine M, Maass AH, et al. Strain imaging to predict response to cardiac resynchronization therapy: a systematic comparison of strain parameters using multiple imaging techniques. ESC Heart Fail. 2018;5(6):1130–40.

52. Kutyifa V, Zareba W, McNitt S, Singh J, Hall WJ, Polonsky S, et al. Left ventricular lead location and the risk of ventricular arrhythmias in the MADIT-CRT trial. Eur Heart J. 2012;34:184–90.

53. Jin Y, Zhang Q, Mao JL, He B. Image-guided left ventricular lead placement in cardiac resynchronization therapy for patients with heart failure: a meta-analysis. BMC Cardiovasc Disord. 2015;15:36.

Chapter 5
Biventricular Pacing for Patients with Complete Heart Block

Hannah E. Wey, Gaurav A. Upadhyay, and Roderick Tung

Introduction and Etiologies of CHB

Complete heart block (CHB), or third-degree atrioventricular block (AVB), is defined by a failure of supraventricular impulses to conduct through the AV node or His bundle. The diagnosis requires that atrial impulses occur at a higher rate than the ventricular rate and that no atrial stimuli lead to ventricular contractions [1]. According to ACC/AHA/HRS guidelines, pacemaker implantation is a class I indication in all patients with advanced second-degree or third-degree AVB who have symptomatic bradycardia, any degree of LV dysfunction, an escape rhythm <40 beats per minute, asystolic pauses >3.0 seconds, or any escape rhythm generated from below the AV node as a means to reduce mortality secondary to sudden cardiac death [2, 3]. The guidelines also specify that it is reasonable (class IIa) to consider permanent pacemaker implantation for persistent third-degree AV block with an escape rate greater than 40 bpm in asymptomatic adult patients without cardiomegaly.

The etiologies of complete heart block are numerous and can be grouped into congenital and acquired AVB (with the latter being significantly more common). Congenital complete atrioventricular block (CCAVB) is a rare entity; it occurs in approximately 1 out of every 15,000–20,000 live births and is mechanistically thought to be due to in utero exposure to maternal antibodies (anti-Ro/SSA and

H. E. Wey
Department of Internal Medicine, University of Chicago Medicine, The Pritzker School of Medicine at the University of Chicago, Chicago, IL, USA

G. A. Upadhyay · R. Tung (✉)
Center for Arrhythmia Care, Heart and Vascular Institute, University of Chicago Medicine, The Pritzker School of Medicine at the University of Chicago, Chicago, IL, USA
e-mail: rodericktung@uchicago.edu

© Springer Nature Switzerland AG 2019
J. S. Steinberg, A. E. Epstein (eds.), *Clinical Controversies in Device Therapy for Cardiac Arrhythmias*, https://doi.org/10.1007/978-3-030-22882-8_5

anti-La/SSB antibodies) leading to inflammatory changes and fibrosis of the conduction system in most cases, although inherited channelopathies may also play a role [4]. It is primarily associated with a junctional escape rhythm and may be associated with a benign clinical course and late diagnosis. Overall mortality, however, in CCAVB without intervention is estimated to be as high as 16% in the neonatal period [5]. Other congenital heart diseases such as hypoplastic left heart syndrome, right and left isomerism, univentricular heart, and L-shaped ventricle are also associated with spontaneous high-degree AVB including complete AVB. The proposed mechanisms include poor coronary supply to both sinoatrial (SA) and atrioventricular (AV) nodes in altered cardiac anatomy with subsequent ischemic damage during the third trimester [6]. Development of a superficial, and perhaps unstable, conduction system is also observed in CHD. CHB may occur due to structural defects within the myocardium such as in AV septal defects or iatrogenically after corrective cardiac surgery.

Acquired complete heart block can occur at any age and can be due to a multitude of causes including iatrogenic, infectious, ischemic, and malignant (see Table 5.1). CHB is a well-accepted indication for permanent pacemaker placement, in both pediatric and adult patients, as well as for the asymptomatic patient who exhibits other signs of high-risk for malignant arrhythmia and sudden cardiac death. This review will discuss the current evidence supporting the use of cardiac resynchronization therapy (CRT) versus conventional right ventricular pacing (RVP) in the setting of CHB.

Table 5.1 Causes of complete heart block

Infectious	Lyme myocarditis
	Chagas myocarditis
	Diphtheric myocarditis
	Rheumatic fever
Inflammatory	Sjogren's syndrome
	Cardiac sarcoidosis
Ischemic	Myocardial infarction
	Aortic dissection
Structural	Post-cardiac surgery
	Post-transcatheter aortic valve insertion/replacement
Malignant	Primary cardiac lymphoma or metastasis
	Head and neck cancers with loss of baroreceptor and/or neurocardiogenic response
Medications	Beta blockers
	Non-dihydropyridine calcium-channel blockers (e.g., verapamil, diltiazem)
	Digoxin
	Clonidine
	Findolamid (used to treat multiple sclerosis)
	Adverse effect of checkpoint inhibitors
Metabolic	Hyperkalemia
	Hypermagnesemia
	Hypothyroidism

Indications for CRT

The 2013 update of ACCF/AHA/HRS practice guidelines for device-based therapy established clear indications for CRT therapy in patients with reduced LVEF, primarily 35%, and symptomatic heart failure (see Table 5.2) [3]. These guidelines were founded on the results of large multicenter randomized controlled trials showing echocardiographic, functional, and mortality benefit when comparing CRT-D to ICD and intrinsic conduction on guideline-directed medical therapy [7–12]; however, these trials did not specifically enroll patients with CHB.

Table 5.2 Indications for cardiac resynchronization therapy (CRT)

Class I	CRT is indicated for patients who have LVEF less than or equal to 35%, sinus rhythm, LBBB with a QRS duration greater than or equal to 150 ms, and NYHA class II, III, or ambulatory IV; symptoms on GDMT (*Level of Evidence: A for NYHA class III/IV; Level of Evidence: B for NYHA class II*)
Class IIa	CRT can be useful for patients who have LVEF less than or equal to 35%, sinus rhythm, LBBB with a QRS duration 120–149 ms, and NYHA class II, III, or ambulatory IV symptoms on GDMT (*Level of Evidence: B*)
	CRT can be useful for patients who have LVEF less than or equal to 35%, sinus rhythm, a non-LBBB pattern with a QRS duration greater than or equal to 150 ms, and NYHA class III/ambulatory class IV symptoms on GDMT (*Level of Evidence: A*)
	CRT can be useful in patients with atrial fibrillation and LVEF less than or equal to 35% on GDMT if (a) the patient requires ventricular pacing or otherwise meets CRT criteria and (b) AV nodal ablation or pharmacologic rate control will allow near 100% ventricular pacing with CRT (*Level of Evidence: B*)
	CRT can be useful for patients on GDMT who have LVEF less than or equal to 35% and are undergoing new or replacement device placement with anticipated requirement for significant (>40%) ventricular pacing (*Level of Evidence: C*)
	In patients with atrioventricular block who have an indication for permanent pacing with an LVEF between 36% and 50% and are expected to require ventricular pacing more than 40% of the time, it is reasonable to choose pacing methods that maintain physiologic ventricular activation (e.g., cardiac resynchronization therapy [CRT] or His bundle pacing) over right ventricular pacing (*Level of Evidence: B-R*) (*new*)
Class IIb	CRT may be considered for patients who have LVEF less than or equal to 30%, ischemic etiology of heart failure, sinus rhythm, LBBB with a QRS duration of greater than or equal to 150 ms, and NYHA class I symptoms on GDMT (*Level of Evidence: C*)
	CRT may be considered for patients who have LVEF less than or equal to 35%, sinus rhythm, a non-LBBB pattern with QRS duration 120–149 ms, and NYHA class III/ambulatory class IV on GDMT (*Level of Evidence: B*)
	CRT may be considered for patients who have LVEF less than or equal to 35%, sinus rhythm, a non-LBBB pattern with a QRS duration greater than or equal to 150 ms, and NYHA class II symptoms on GDMT (*Level of Evidence: B*)
Class III	CRT is not recommended for patients with NYHA class I or II symptoms and non-LBBB pattern with QRS duration less than 150 ms (*Level of Evidence: B*)
	CRT is not indicated for patients whose comorbidities and/or frailty limit survival with good functional capacity to less than 1 year (*Level of Evidence: C*)

Outside the realm of sinus rhythm, the 2013 practice guidelines make a class IIa recommendation for CRT in patients with atrial fibrillation and LVEF ≤35% on guideline-directed medical therapy who otherwise meet criteria for CRT implantation as well as for those with atrial fibrillation who have received AV nodal ablation or pharmacologic rate control requiring near 100% ventricular pacing [3]. The recently released 2018 ACC/AHA/HRS guidelines on the evaluation and management of patients with bradycardia and cardiac conduction delay also provide a class IIa recommendation for consideration for CRT or His bundle pacing in patients with LVEF between 36% and 50% who are anticipated to receive >40% ventricular pacing [2].

CRT in Heart Failure with Reduced Ejection Fraction (LVEF ≤35%)

While multiple studies have been performed in CRT in patients with heart failure, there have only been two randomized controlled trials (RCTs) conducted to date comparing RVP with CRT in the setting of reduced LVEF. The 2006 Homburg Biventricular Pacing Evaluation (HOBIPACE) trial was the first trial to address RVP versus CRT in patients with a standard antibradycardia indication [13]. The study was a single-center, single-blind, prospective RCT of 30 patients with LVEF <40% and LV end-diastolic diameter ≥60 mm with NYHA class III–IV symptoms on optimal medical management. The enrolled population had an average LVEF of 26% and an average QRS duration of 174 ms. All patients received atrio-biventricular devices and were randomized to either RVP or CRT and received 3 months of therapy prior to crossing over to the other pacing mode. Primary endpoints measured were LVEF, left ventricular end-systolic volume (LVESV), and peak oxygen consumption. Secondary endpoints measured were NYHA functional class, quality of life as assessed by questionnaire, and serum concentration of N-terminal pro-B-type natriuretic peptide (NT-proBNP).

When compared with RVP, patients receiving CRT showed significantly reduced LVESV (17% decline), significantly increased LVEF (22% rise), and significantly increased peak oxygen consumption (12% increase) during biventricular stimulation. Secondary endpoints of left ventricular end diastolic volume (LVEDV) and NT-proBNP were also significantly reduced in the CRT compared with RVP. They also found other measures of favorable LV remodeling, including significant decrease in LV mass and subsequent increase in hypertrophy index in CRT as compared to RVP. No difference in mortality was found, although the study was underpowered for this endpoint.

Patients with atrial fibrillation and AVB were included in HOBIPACE. Over one-third (11 or 37%) of patients demonstrated AF at enrollment, with 9 patients who continued to be in permanent atrial fibrillation throughout the course of the study. Subgroup analysis of AF patients did not show any difference in echocardiographic or clinical outcomes compared to those in sinus rhythm. Taken together, the results of HOBIPACE provided compelling support of CRT over traditional RVP in those with reduced LVEF and prolonged QRS duration; however, this study did not evaluate patients with high-degree AVB [13].

The only other RCT evaluating CRT versus RVP in patients with reduced LVEF is the 2010 Conventional Versus Biventricular Pacing in Heart Failure and Bradyarrhythmia (COMBAT) trial [14]. This study was a multicenter, prospective, double-blind crossover study of 60 patients. Patients enrolled had an average LVEF of 29–30%, QRS duration of 148–154 ms, and NYHA class II–IV symptoms. Fifty percent of all patients had CHB in this study. Patients underwent a minimum of 3-month intervals of RVP/CRT/RVP pacing or CRT/RVP/CRT pacing modalities and were ultimately followed for 17.5 months. Primary endpoints evaluated were quality of life as assessed by the Minnesota Living with Heart Failure Questionnaire and NYHA functional class. Secondary endpoints were 6-min walk test, peak oxygen consumption during cardiopulmonary exercise, echocardiographic parameters, and mortality.

Patients receiving biventricular stimulation in COMBAT showed significant improvement in all primary endpoints at the end of each crossover period, as well as LVEF and LVESV. There was no significant difference between modalities in 6-min walk test or peak oxygen consumption. Of the 25% of patients who died during the study period, they were significantly more likely to be in a RVP period than during CRT period. COMBAT did not include patients in atrial fibrillation (in contrast to HOBIPACE), had stricter LV lead placement requirements, and was double-blind compared to single-blind design. Although also small in comparison the landmark trials that led to the approval of CRT for primary prevention indications, COMBAT showed supportive data, particularly with respect to echocardiographic and clinical parameters—that a biventricular pacing mode was superior to RVP in patients with high-degree AVB and reduced LVEF (see Table 5.3).

More recently, a nonrandomized study examining the role of CRT in patients with heart block and low LVEF was conducted by Shimano and colleagues in 2007 [15]. They sought to evaluate the treatment of patients with RV pacing-induced cardiomyopathy and evaluated 18 patients with acquired CHB who had received RVP and subsequently developed pacemaker-induced cardiomyopathy and heart failure. The average LVEF at the time of upgrade was 28%, whereas the original LVEF at the time of device placement was 54%. Patients had received a mean of 81 months of RVP prior to upgrade. This study followed patients for 12 months after device upgrade from RVP to CRT-D or LV-ICD devices. The results of this study showed significantly improved LVEF (28% to 34%), NYHA functional class (mean 3.0–1.9), as well as reduced LV end-diastolic diameter, left atrial diameter, mitral regurgitation severity, and serum BNP level. Heart failure hospitalization rate per year was also significantly reduced after upgrade to CRT from 2.1 per year to 0.3 per year [15].

CRT in Patients with Preserved Ejection Fraction (LVEF ≥50%)

To date, there have been three RCTs that have evaluated the role of CRT compared with RVP in patients with preserved LVEF. The first was the Pacing to Avoid Cardiac Enlargement (PACE) trial in 2009 [16]. A multicenter, prospective, double-blind

Table 5.3 Randomized controlled trials evaluating cardiac resynchronization therapy in patients with high-degree AV block and heart failure with reduced ejection fraction (≤35%)

Clinical trial or study	Study design	Population	QRS duration (mean)	LVEF (mean)	Summary of findings
HOBIPACE (2006)	Single-center, prospective, single-blinded RCT Crossover comparison of RV and BiV pacing of patients with symptomatic bradycardia requiring permanent pacemaker Followed for 6 months: 3 months of each pacing modality	N = 30 patients Mean age 69.7 years old NYHA class III–IV, LVEF <40%, and LVEDD ≥60 mm Included atrial fibrillation patients (11/30 patients)	174 ms	26%	Significantly lower LVEDV, LVESV, and NT-proBNP in BiV group Significantly higher LVEF, cardiac index, and peak O2 consumption in BiV group Improved exercise capacity and quality of life in BiV group
COMBAT (2010)	Multicenter, prospective, double-blind RCT Crossover study of RVP versus BiV pacing in those with AV block as an indication for pacing Followed for average of 17.5 months, minimum of 3 months in each pacing modality	N = 60 patients: 31 patients underwent RVP/BiV/RVP, 29 patients underwent BiV/RVP/BiV Mean ages 57.4/59.3 years old NYHA class II–IV, LVEF ≤40%, and on optimal medical therapy for 30 days Excluded atrial fibrillation patients	148 ms (RVP) 154 ms (BiV) 15/31 and 15/29 patients in each arm had complete heart block	29% (RVP) and 30% (BiV)	Significant improvement in quality of life, NYHA class, LVEF, and LVESV with BiV pacing 15/60 (25%) patients died. Of these, significantly more were in an RVP period

trial, PACE enrolled 177 patients with symptomatic bradycardia and preserved LVEF ≥45% (average LVEF 62%) and randomized patients to conventional RV apical pacing or CRT. The original study followed patients for 12 months [16], and a 24-month follow-up was subsequently published in 2011 [17]. The average QRS duration was 107 ms, and approximately 50–60% of patients had advanced AVB as indication for pacemaker placement. Primary endpoints evaluated were LVEF and LVESV.

After 24 months, LVEF significantly decreased in the RVP group (62–53%), and this was also a significant difference when compared to patients receiving biventricular pacing, who demonstrated preservation of LVEF over the study period (62–63%). Similarly, LVESV significantly increased in RVP (28.4–38.3 mL over

24 months) and also was significantly increased compared to CRT (28.2–25.3 mL over 24 months). However, there were no significant differences in clinical measures such as heart failure hospitalizations, mortality, or quality of life between groups [16, 17]. Although the results of PACE argue in favor of biventricular pacing to protect LVEF and structural parameters, this did not translate to clinical outcomes during the studied period in patients with preserved LVEF and a narrow QRS complex at baseline.

Shortly after PACE, the authors of the Preventing Ventricular Dysfunction in Pacemaker Patients Without Advanced Heart Failure (PREVENT-HF) trial reported similar findings 2 years later. PREVENT-HF was an international multicenter, prospective, single-blind study of 108 patients with normal LVEF undergoing device implant for AV block which randomized patients to receive either DDD-R dual-chamber RV apical pacing or biventricular pacing systems. This trial selected patients with class I or IIa indication for permanent pacemaker and with an anticipated overall pacing rate of ≥80%. The groups were well-matched, with no significant differences in LVEF (55% RVP versus 58% CRT), QRS duration (121 ms RVP versus 124 ms CRT), and other basic demographics including gender and major comorbidities. Patients were randomized to RV apical pacing or biventricular pacing strategies and followed for 12 months. Of note, however, there was significant crossover due to inability to implant an LV lead affecting 16% of the patients assigned to biventricular pacing. The primary endpoint measured was change in LVEDV, and secondary endpoints evaluated were LVESV, LVEF, mitral regurgitation, and clinical composite of heart failure events or cardiovascular hospitalization. This trial showed no significant difference in any of the outcomes measured in patients with high degree of ventricular pacing and preserved LVEF, although the authors noted that follow-up time was short and that small numeric improvement in LVEF (but not reaching statistical significance) was noted in patients receiving biventricular pacing in the on-treatment analysis [18].

Most recently, the Biventricular Pacing for Atrioventricular Block to Prevent Cardiac Desynchronization (BioPace) study was performed and preliminary data released in 2014, although the final manuscript remains unpublished. BioPace was a large, multicenter, prospective, single-blind RCT enrolling 1,810 patients, and its findings with respect to the impact of biventricular pacing has been highly anticipated. Enrollment criteria were broad, including patients NYHA class I–III symptoms irrespective of LVEF. The most important requirement was AV block and anticipated need for ventricular pacing ≥67% of the time. BioPace included patients with atrial tachyarrhythmias (24% of patients). Of these patients, 400 (22%) had CHB, and an additional 573 (32%) had intermittent CHB or type II second-degree AVB. Patients were then randomized to RV versus biventricular pacing systems and followed for an average of 5.6 years. Baseline QRS duration overall was 119 ms. LVEF overall in all patients was 55%; if further broken down, 1239/1810 (68%) of patients had LVEF >50%; of these, the average LVEF was 62% [19].

The primary endpoint assessed in BioPace was a combined clinical endpoint of time to death and time to first heart failure hospitalization. The preliminary analysis

showed no significant difference in the primary outcome between RVP and biventricular pacing strategies; this remained true even substratifying based on LVEF
>50% and LVEF ≤50% subgroups [20]. Since the final manuscript has not been
published, we do not have data regarding if there were subgroups of benefit with
CRT, such as those with higher-degree RV pacing or high-degree AV block. At this
point, however, the results are not suggestive of uniform benefit of CRT in patients
with normal LVEF.

Taken together, three RCTs, BioPace, PREVENT-HF, and PACE, all resulted in
no difference in hard clinical outcomes for patients who received CRT versus RVP
with preserved LVEF (see Table 5.4) as a de novo strategy. This is an interesting
contrast with studies like Shimano's which show that—for patients with normal
LVEF at baseline who develop RV pacing-induced cardiomyopathy after months or
years of pacing—biventricular upgrade is a reasonable treatment approach. These
findings suggest that the population of patients with normal LVEF at baseline and
anticipated need for high-degree of RV pacing is heterogenous and that we must
investigate other possible indicators or signals of risk prior to upfront biventricular
pacing.

More recent registry data from Merchant et al. investigated 21,202 patients, of
whom close to one-third had a documented history of complete heart block [21].
They found that patients with preexisting complete heart block were more likely to
demonstrate a new diagnosis of heart failure in follow-up than patients without this
diagnosis (and therefore likely receiving less RV pacing). With respect to predictors
of heart failure, they found that younger age (≤55 years old) and history of atrial
fibrillation were significant predictors of both increased heart failure early (within
6 months) and late (between 6 months and 4 years) after device implant. An important limitation of this study, however, is that baseline LVEF and pacing burden were
not retrievable, and therefore interpretation with respect to patient selection remains
limited from these large registry data.

CRT in Patients with Intermediate Ejection Fraction (LVEF 36–49%)

In patients with intermediate LVEF, there have been two RCTs that have evaluated
the role of RVP versus biventricular pacing. The first of these is the Left Ventricular-
Based Cardiac Stimulation Post AV Nodal Ablation Evaluation (PAVE) study,
which was published in 2005 [22]. PAVE was a multicenter, prospective, single-
blind RCT of 184 patients who were to receive AV nodal ablation for chronic atrial
fibrillation with rapid ventricular response refractory to medical management. This
post-AV nodal ablation population was targeted given the need for post-ablation
pacemaker placement and the inference that patients would be primarily reliant on
ventricular pacing for nearly 100% of ventricular beats. Patients with NYHA class
II–III symptoms and no previous pacemaker or implantable cardioverter-defibrillator

Table 5.4 Randomized controlled trials evaluating cardiac resynchronization in patients with high degree AV block and preserved ejection fraction (EF ≥50%)

Clinical trial or study	Study design	Population	QRS duration (mean)	LVEF (mean)	Summary of findings
PACE (2009)	Multicenter, prospective, double-blind RCT of patients with indication for primary pacemaker and preserved ejection fraction. BiV or RVP pacing. Followed for 12 months in original study. Follow up study performed at 24 months	N = 177. 89 patients in BiV pacing group, 88 patients in RVP group. Mean age 68–69 years old. Indication for PPM: SND, high-degree AVB. LVEF≥45%. Excluded if in persistent AF, unstable angina, ACS, or PCI/CABG within previous 3 months. Included patients with permanent AF	107 ms. 55/88 had advanced AVB in RVP group. 49/89 had advanced AVB in CRT group	62%	Significantly lower LVEF and higher LVESV in RVP group. LVEF and LVESV unchanged in BiV pacing group. No difference in death, HF hospitalization, or QOL assessment
PREVENT-HF (2011)	Multicenter, prospective, single-blind RCT of patients with normal LVEF and class I or IIa indication for PPM with need for ventricular pacing ≥80% of the time. Followed for 12 months	N = 108. 58 patients in RVP and 50 patients in CRT. Mean age 70–72 years old. Excluded NYHA class III–IV, MI, or cardiac surgery in previous 3 months, hypertrophic cardiomyopathy, or previous device	121 ms in RVP group. 124 ms in CRT group. 13/58 patients in RVP and 10/50 patients in CRT were dependent on PPM inferring high-degree AVB	55% in RVP group. 58% in CRT group	Followed for 12 months: no significant difference in LVEDV, LVEF, LVESV, development or worsening MR, heart failure symptoms, cardiac mortality, or hospitalization
BioPace (2014)	Multicenter, prospective, single-blind RCT of 1810 patients with high-degree AV block requiring >67% ventricular pacing and NYHA class I–III symptoms comparing RVP versus BiV pacing. Mean follow up 5.6 years	N = 1810. 902 patients in BiV, 908 patients in RVP. Mean age 74 years old. LBBB present in 17% of patients overall, 24% with atrial tachyarrhythmia	119 ms overall. 400/1810 patients were indicated for complete heart block. 573/1810 patients were indicated for intermittent third-degree AV block or type II second-degree heart block with prolonged PR interval	55% overall. 1239/1810 patients with LVEF >50%. Of these, mean EF 61.9%	No significant difference in combined endpoint of time to death and time to first heart failure hospitalization, which remained nonsignificant despite subgroup analysis by LVEF ≤50% and LVEF >50%

(ICD) were included. Baseline LVEF was 46%. Patients were then randomized to receive either a conventional RVP device or a biventricular device and subsequently underwent AV nodal ablation within the following 4 weeks. Notably, 146 patients were originally randomized to the CRT group; however, 23 patients were lost to follow-up and 21 patients were withdrawn due to failed LV lead placement. Comparatively, 106 patients were randomized to the RVP group, of which 25 were lost to follow-up, but all device implantation procedures were completed successfully. This again highlights the technical difficulty of biventricular placement over traditional dual-chamber devices [22]. Patients were followed for 6 months' duration.

The primary endpoint studied in PAVE was 6-min walk test distance before and after the study period. Secondary endpoints included quality of life as assessed by SF-36 Health Status Scale survey and LVEF. Compared to RVP, patients who received CRT had significantly improved 6-min walk distance (31% improvement from baseline compared to 24% improvement in RVP group). This change was primarily driven by patients with LVEF ≤45%, and in further subgroup analysis, 6-min walk distance was not significantly different between pacing modalities in patients with LVEF >45%. Additionally, LVEF remained unchanged at 6 months in the CRT group, but LVEF significantly decreased in the RVP group (46–41%). There was no significant difference in quality of life at 6 months post-ablation, even when further broken down by NYHA functional class, nor was there a significant difference in mortality between groups. Thus, PAVE showed evidence of clinical improvement as determined by 6-min walk distance in patients with LVEF ≤45% in favor of CRT over RVP as well as relative preservation of LVEF. However, this did not translate to a significant mortality benefit (although the trial was underpowered to show this), and it is clear that the favorable outcomes for CRT patients were driven by those with clinical heart failure and lower LVEF at baseline.

Following PAVE, which was specific to post-AV nodal ablation patients with refractory atrial fibrillation, the landmark Biventricular Pacing for Atrioventricular Block and Systolic Dysfunction (BLOCK HF) Trial was published in 2013 [23]. BLOCK HF was a multicenter, prospective, double-blind RCT of 691 patients with mild-moderate heart failure and high degree of ventricular pacing. Patients were included with third-degree AVB (with 47% enrolled with CHB), advanced second-degree AVB, or first-degree AVB with PR interval ≥300 ms when paced at 100 bpm and LVEF ≤50% with NYHA class I–III symptoms. The study also included patients with permanent atrial fibrillation and those undergoing AV nodal ablation. Importantly, 207 patients received ICD placement as well. Patients were randomized to CRT or RVP and followed for an average of 37 months [23]. BLOCK HF demonstrated significant technical difficulty with device implantation in which 113/809 patients in whom device implantation was attempted had a serious adverse effect within the first 30 days after implantation, of which 83 patients had complications related to the implantation procedure or the CRT device itself. Adverse events included lead dislodgement, lead damage, failure to capture, implantation site infection, and atrial fibrillation.

The primary endpoint studied in BLOCK-HF was time to death of any cause, an urgent care visit for heart failure requiring intravenous medical therapy, or a ≥15% increase in LVESV index. Secondary endpoints included two clinical composite outcomes: urgent care visit for heart failure or death of any cause and heart failure hospitalization or death of any cause. The primary endpoint occurred significantly more in the RVP group compared to the CRT group with a hazard ratio of 0.74, which remained consistent between those with and without ICD placement. Similarly, when LVESV index information was removed, the primary endpoint of time to death of any cause or an urgent care visit for heart failure significantly favored CRT over RVP. The composite secondary endpoints and time to first heart failure hospitalization were significantly less in the CRT group compared to RVP, although all-cause mortality was not significantly different between groups.

A subgroup of the previously discussed BioPace trial had intermediate LVEF (41%). This subgroup was comprised of 571/1810 (32%) patients [20]. When analyzed separately, this group similarly did not show a significant difference in the primary outcome of combined time to death and time to first heart failure hospitalization. The results of BioPace, BLOCK HF, and PAVE have conflicting results in regard to clinical outcomes of CRT versus RVP in patients with intermediate LVEF (Table 5.5). Where BLOCK HF and PAVE found evidence of at least some degree of clinical improvement with CRT over traditional RV apical pacing in patients with CHB or advanced AVB, BioPace, the largest RCT conducted to date on this population, did not find a significant difference, although it remains unpublished. The 2018 bradycardia guidelines, however, have incorporated the results of BLOCK-HF, and biventricular pacing (or His bundle pacing) may be considered (class IIa indication) in patients receiving device therapy with an anticipated >40% pacing and an LVEF of 36–50%.

Congenital Heart Block

CHD and CCAVB are a special patient population with a unique array of clinical features. Many infants with CCAVB or other structural cardiac abnormalities will require pacemaker placement with or without ICD placement due to symptomatic bradycardia, progressive LV dysfunction, malignant arrhythmia or as primary prevention. Although there are no randomized controlled trials comparing traditional RVP and biventricular pacing, in this population, several case reports and case series do exist in the literature (see Table 5.6) which suggest that biventricular pacing may be of benefit.

A multicenter cross-sectional study of 178 children with structurally normal hearts, advanced second-degree or third-degree AVB, and >70% ventricular pacing requirement was conducted by Janousek et al. and published in 2013. Notably, 171/178 patients had CHB, and 138/178 patients had CCAVB. Patients underwent ventricular pacemaker placement at various locations including RVOT, RV lateral wall, RV septum, RV apex, LV basal wall, LV lateral wall, and LV apex. Patients

Table 5.5 Randomized controlled trials evaluating cardiac resynchronization in patients with high-degree AV block and intermediate ejection fraction (36–49%)

Clinical trial or study	Study design	Population	QRS duration (mean)	LVEF (mean)	Summary of findings
PAVE (2005)	Multicenter, prospective, single-blind RCT of patients undergoing AVN ablation for chronic AF with RVR refractory to medical therapy with subsequent pacemaker implantation: BiV device or RVP device Followed for 6 months	N = 184 103 patients in BiV groups, 81 patients in RVP group Mean age 67 years old in RVP, 70 years old in BiV group NYHA class II–III symptoms Excluded NYHA class IV, required ICD, cardiac surgery, or prosthetic valve present		46%	Significantly improved 6-min walk distance in BiV group, driven by those with LVEF ≤45% No significant difference in 6-min walk distance between groups when LVEF >45% Significant drop in LVEF in RVP group, which was avoided in BiV group No significant difference in quality of life assessment
BLOCK-HF (2013)	Multicenter, prospective, double-blind RCT comparing RVP to CRT in patients with mild-moderate heart failure, LVEF≤50%, and high degree of ventricular pacing High degree of ventricular pacing defined as: third-degree AV block, advanced second-degree block, or first-degree block with PR interval ≥300 ms when paced at 100 bpm (class I or IIa indication for PPM) NYHA class I–III symptoms and LVEF ≤50% Included patients with permanent atrial arrhythmias and post-AVN ablation Followed for average of 37 months	N = 691 patients: 346 in CRT, 342 in RVP 13 crossed over from BiV to RVP 84 crossed over from RVP to BiV 207 received ICD, 484 did not have ICD 97.0–98.6% ventricular pacing Mean age 73 years old	123 ms (RVP) 124 ms (CRT) 47% of all patients had third-degree AV block	40%	Primary endpoint: time to an urgent care visit for HF requiring IV therapy, time to all-cause mortality, or ≥15% increase in LVESV index significantly improved in CRT group Secondary endpoints: composite outcome of heart failure hospitalization or death and time to first HF hospitalization significantly improved in CRT group over RVP in both ICD and pacemaker groups
BioPace (2014)	Multicenter, prospective, single-blind RCT of 1810 patients, design outlined previously	N = 1810	119 ms overall	571/1810 patients with LVEF ≤50%: of which mean EF 41%	No significant difference in combined endpoint of time to death and time to first heart failure hospitalization, which remained nonsignificant despite subgroup analysis by LVEF ≤50% and LVEF >50%

Table 5.6 Studies evaluating cardiac resynchronization therapy in congenital heart disease with high-degree AV block

Study name	Study design and population	QRS duration (mean)	LVEF (mean)	Summary of findings
Janousek et al. (2013)	Multicenter cross-sectional study of 178 children with structurally normal hearts and indication for PPM: second- or third-degree heart block with predicted >70% ventricular pacing Median age at implantation: 3.2 years old Median pacing duration 5.4 years	171/178 patients had complete heart block 138/178 patients had congenital CHB	Pre-implantation: all groups >60% Post-implantation: RVP: 53%, LVP 60%	Significant drop in LVEF and LV shortening fraction in all RV pacing and LV basal pacing sites; no significant drop in LVEF or LV shortening fraction in LV apical or LV lateral wall pacing Observable dyssynchrony by ECHO in RVOT and RV lateral wall pacing compared to other pacing sites RV septum not significantly improved compared to other RV pacing sites LV basal pacing inferior to LV apex and LV lateral wall Maternal antibodies not a predictor of LV dysfunction
Motonaga and Dubin (2014)	Systematic review of CRT in pediatric patients with HF and CHD 7 single-center and 2 multi-center retrospective studies of HF in CHD	166 ms in multicenter reviews 66/101 of patients from single-center studies with complete AVB	26–27% in multicenter reviews	All studies found an increase in LVEF and decreased QRS duration 10–30% nonresponder rate, defined as no change in NYHA or <10% improvement in LVEF, among these reviews

were followed for a median of 5.4 years. This study observed a significant decrease in LVEF in all RV pacing sites and LV basal pacing compared to LV lateral wall and LV apical pacing sites with the most subjective ventricular dyssynchrony occurring at RVOT and RV lateral wall sites [24]. Although not specifically engaged in CRT, this study supports the concept that worsening ventricular dyssynchrony by non-physiologic cardiac conduction, even in children with structurally normal hearts and preserved LVEF, is deleterious compared to synchronous ventricular contraction.

In 2014, Motonaga and Dubin conducted a systematic review of CRT in CHD and associated heart failure. This review incorporated seven single-center studies and two multicenter retrospective studies. This review specifically identified 66/101 patients to have complete AVB. Prior to implantation, baseline QRS was 166 ms in the multicenter reviews, and baseline LVEF was 26%. All studies found increased LVEF after CRT implantation and narrowed QRS complex compared to baseline [25]. Although CRT was not compared to any other form of pacing in these studies, it may provide one of several non-pharmacologic therapies for pediatric patients with CHD and heart failure with or without complete AVB.

Post-AV Nodal Ablation

In addition to the findings of the PAVE trial (2005), a large retrospective observational cohort study using the MarketScan Commercial and Medicare supplemental claims database was performed regarding patients with atrial fibrillation who underwent AV junction ablation (AVJA) followed by pacemaker implantation [26]. The study included 24,361 patients, of which 1611 underwent AVJA, 23,377 received RVP, and 984 received biventricular pacemakers. The study compared risk of hospitalization due to atrial fibrillation between AVJA and non-AVJA groups, finding a significant reduction in the AVJA group (hazard ratio 0.31). They also compared risk of heart failure hospitalization in CRT versus RVP and found a significant increase in risk in patients who received RVP after AVJA compared to non-AVJA (hazard ratio 1.63), whereas no-such increased risk occurred in those who received CRT after AVJA.

Another prospective, double-blind, multicenter, randomized controlled trial of 186 patients by Brignole and colleagues in 2011 compared patients who had undergone AVJA for symptomatic permanent atrial fibrillation who then received biventricular pacing versus traditional RVP [27]. Average LVEF at enrollment was 38% in the CRT group ($N = 97$) and 37% in the RVP group ($N = 89$). 40% of patients received ICD placement as well in both groups, and 50% of patients in both groups had baseline QRS $\geq$120 ms. Patients were followed for a median of 20 months with crossover due to clinical failure as defined by the primary endpoint of composite HF hospitalization, death due to HF, or clinically worsening HF. This study found a statistically significant reduction in the primary endpoint in those who received CRT over RVP primarily driven by reduction in HF hospitalization and clinically worsening HF. All-cause mortality was similar between groups.

In patients with LVEF ≤35%, QRS ≥120 ms, and NYHA class ≥III–IV, which represented 25% of study patients and the population indicated for CRT by both American and European guidelines, there was a significant clinical decline as defined by incidence of the primary outcome in RVP as compared to CRT. Interestingly, among the 75% of patients who did not meet the above criteria, the statistical significance of clinical performance remained present favoring CRT over RVP.

Discussion

It has been well-established that nonreversible CHB is usually an unstable bradyarrhythmia that requires pacemaker support. Overall, there are limited data directly comparing RVP versus biventricular pacing with an LV lead in patients receiving devices for high-degree AV block. We believe that the available data suggest that a tailored approach of selecting RV versus biventricular pacing should be pursued based on underlying LVEF, pacing burden, and clinical scenario.

In patients with CHB and reduced LVEF ≤35%, evidence from two prospective, randomized trials—HOBIPACE and COMBAT—along with data from multiple cohort studies, consistently show echocardiographic and clinical improvement in CRT over traditional RV apical pacing. Improved LVEF (see Fig. 5.1), LV dimensions, cardiac index, exercise capacity, and quality-of-life scores were observed among these trials. These findings may correlate with the degree of ventricular dyssynchrony and prolonged QRS duration documented in both studies, with average-paced QRS dura-

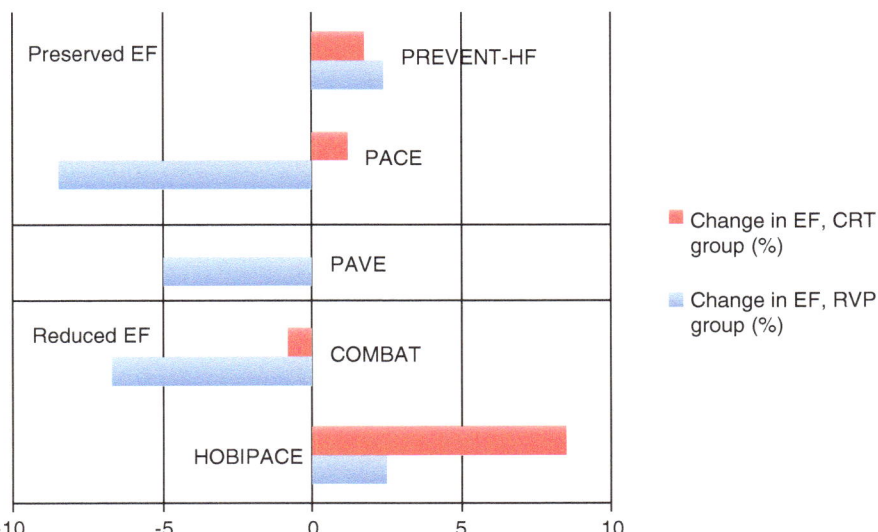

Fig. 5.1 Comparison of change in ejection fraction between RVP and CRT groups in randomized controlled studies

tions greater than 150 ms. It has also been well documented that RVP leads to an abnormal LV electrical activation sequence and functional LBBB and thus may lead to inefficient ventricular contraction and worsening LVEF over time even in patients with previously normal LVEF [28, 29]. It is thought that this abnormal electrical activation predisposes to increased mechanical work at the level of myocardial fibers with increased oxygen consumption [30–32]. The benefit of CRT in patients with reduced LVEF and prolonged QRS duration independent of AVB has also been demonstrated as well [33]. Given the consistency of data showing clinical improvement in patients with high-degree AVB and significant systolic dysfunction (≤35% at baseline), CRT is the most appropriate choice in this population.

In patients with preserved LVEF, however, the current data do not support *routine* selection of CRT over RVP. BioPace and PREVENT-HF found no significant differences in clinical or echocardiographic parameters between RVP and CRT groups. PACE found preservation of LVEF in CRT compared to RVP, but again this study showed no evidence of significant clinical change within the study time frame. More recent large registry data of patients with AVJA suggest that biventricular pacing is associated with less heart failure hospitalization, but data on remodeling or LVEF is unavailable [26]. Importantly, implantation of a left ventricular lead is a technically more advanced procedure and is associated with a higher rate of complications than traditional RVP. In 2012, the European Heart Rhythm Association/HRS expert consensus reported 5–9% implantation failure and 3–7% coronary sinus lead dislodgement [34]. Therefore, without clinical benefit and elevated procedural risk, the current data do not support the routine use of CRT over traditional RVP in patients with CHB and preserved LVEF. Nonetheless, patients should be closely followed with attending to the development of pacemaker-induced cardiomyopathy given the degree of ventricular pacing required in complete AVB. In patients who develop pacing-induced dysfunction, CRT upgrade is a reasonable approach. Not focused on this chapter, His bundle pacing (HBP) may also be another means of addressing pacing-induced cardiomyopathy and is under current study [35].

Device selection should be tailored more carefully in patients with intermediate LVEF and CHB. While BLOCK-HF (average LVEF of 40%) was a positive study and showed significant improvement in combined clinical outcomes with CRT over RVP, a subgroup of BioPace found no change in clinical outcomes between pacing modalities (although rates of pacing have yet to be reported). PAVE additionally found echocardiographic improvement with CRT and maintenance of LVEF but was driven by patients with lower LVEFs. CRT implantation can be considered in this population depending on implantation risk, comorbidities, and risk of development of pacemaker-induced cardiomyopathy. There is a growing consideration for use of HBP in this population. Randomized controlled trials are ongoing to assess efficacy and safety of HBP compared with LV and biventricular devices. A systematic review of HBP cases from 26 articles and 1438 patients with baseline intermediate LVEF (average 43%) found an 84.8% successful implantation rate with improvement in LVEF by 6% [35]. HBP may be a future pacing modality with improved implantation rates and perhaps less operative risk in this population.

The same concepts are seen in the limited data on post-AV nodal ablation and CHD patients. Often these patients will also have reduced LVEF and other structural abnormalities present, and patients with CCAVB and CHD appear to clinically benefit from CRT. Although there are no RCT data to prove the benefit of CRT or LV pacing over traditional RVP, the limited data of case reports and case series show that there is clinical benefit from ventricular resynchrony particularly in those with a wide QRS and visualized dyssynchrony. In post-AVJA patients, CRT appears to benefit these patients over traditional RVP in terms of preserving LVEF and reducing clinical progression of HF and HF hospitalization. PAVE along with studies by Brignole and Mittal et al. found a drop in LVEF in RVP after AV nodal ablation as compared to biventricular pacing. Clinically, Mittal and colleagues found a relative reduction in heart failure hospitalizations in patients with CRT compared to those with RVP, but baseline LVEF was unavailable. Meanwhile, Brignole and colleagues found a reduction in clinical worsening of HF and HF hospitalizations in patients who received CRT as compared to RVP; although the average LVEF in this study was reduced, 60% of patients had intermediate or preserved EF. It is unclear, therefore, whether CRT after AVJA would benefit all patients universally, irrespective of LVEF, although physiologically maintaining some degree of synchrony (with biventricular pacing or HBP) remains the most attractive option.

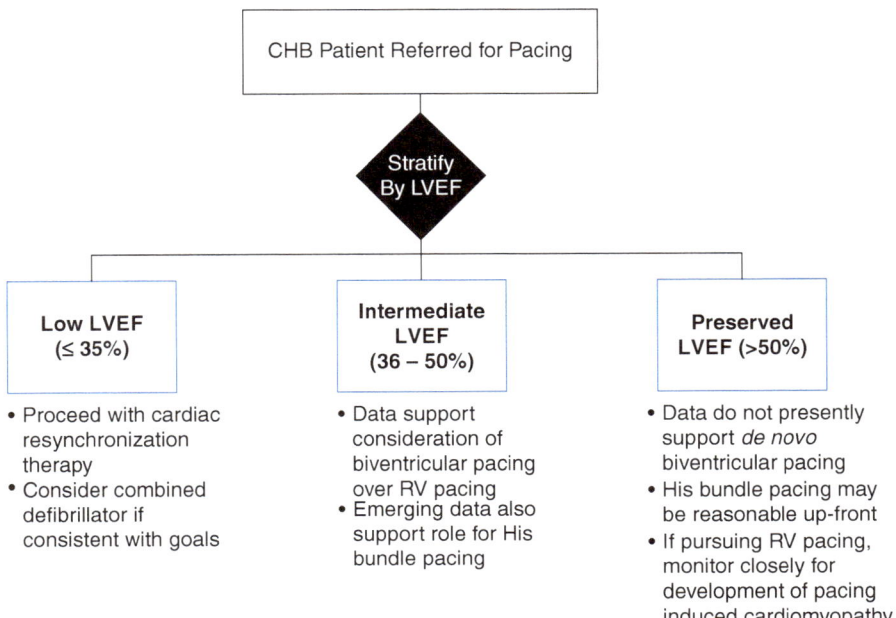

Fig. 5.2 Suggested decision tree for device selection in patients with complete heart block

Conclusion

The weight of the evidence supports the use of CRT in patients with reduced LVEF, is likely beneficial in those with intermediate LVEF, but should not be routinely pursued in patients with preserved LVEF, particularly due to higher perioperative risk and due to the technical difficulty of implanting an LV lead in a minority of patients. A suggested approach is outlined in Fig. 5.2. Future research should focus on better risk stratifying patients at risk for RV pacing-induced cardiomyopathy beyond baseline LVEF, particularly with respect to underlying biomarkers or genetic predisposition to structural or functional decline. In addition, alternative site pacing, including His bundle pacing and conduction system pacing, should also be considered as a complement or alternative to biventricular pacing.

References

1. Vogler J, Breithardt G, Eckardt L. Bradyarrhythmias and conduction blocks. Rev Esp Cardiol (Engl Ed). 2012;65(7):656–67.
2. Kusumoto FM, Schoenfeld MH, Barrett C, Edgerton JR, Ellenbogen KA, Gold MR, Goldschlager NF, Hamilton RM, Joglar JA, Kim RJ, Lee R, Marine JE, McLeod CJ, Oken KR, Patton KK, Pellegrini CN, Selzman KA, Thompson A, Varosy PD. 2018 ACC/AHA/HRS guideline on the evaluation and management of patients with bradycardia and cardiac conduction delay: executive summary: a report of the American College of Cardiology/American Heart Association Task Force on Clinical Practice Guidelines, and the Heart Rhythm Society. J Am Coll Cardiol. 2019.
3. Epstein AE, DiMarco JP, Ellenbogen KA, et al. 2012 ACCF/AHA/HRS focused update incorporated into the ACCF/AHA/HRS 2008 guidelines for device-based therapy of cardiac rhythm abnormalities: a report of the American College of Cardiology Foundation/American Heart Association Task Force on Practice Guidelines and the Heart Rhythm Society. Circulation. 2013;127(3):e283–352.
4. Clancy RM, Kapur RP, Molad Y, Askanase AD, Buyon JP. Immunohistologic evidence supports apoptosis, IgG deposition, and novel macrophage/fibroblast crosstalk in the pathologic cascade leading to congenital heart block. Arthritis Rheum. 2004;50(1):173–82.
5. Baruteau AE, Pass RH, Thambo JB, et al. Congenital and childhood atrioventricular blocks: pathophysiology and contemporary management. Eur J Pediatr. 2016;175(9):1235–48.
6. Ho SY, Esscher E, Anderson RH, Michaelsson M. Anatomy of congenital complete heart block and relation to maternal anti-Ro antibodies. Am J Cardiol. 1986;58(3):291–4.
7. Abraham WT, Fisher WG, Smith AL, et al. Cardiac resynchronization in chronic heart failure. N Engl J Med. 2002;346(24):1845–53.
8. Cleland JG, Daubert JC, Erdmann E, et al. The effect of cardiac resynchronization on morbidity and mortality in heart failure. N Engl J Med. 2005;352(15):1539–49.
9. Bristow MR, Saxon LA, Boehmer J, et al. Cardiac-resynchronization therapy with or without an implantable defibrillator in advanced chronic heart failure. N Engl J Med. 2004;350(21):2140–50.
10. Moss AJ, Hall WJ, Cannom DS, et al. Cardiac-resynchronization therapy for the prevention of heart-failure events. N Engl J Med. 2009;361(14):1329–38.
11. Tang AS, Wells GA, Talajic M, et al. Cardiac-resynchronization therapy for mild-to-moderate heart failure. N Engl J Med. 2010;363(25):2385–95.

12. Linde C, Abraham WT, Gold MR, et al. Randomized trial of cardiac resynchronization in mildly symptomatic heart failure patients and in asymptomatic patients with left ventricular dysfunction and previous heart failure symptoms. J Am Coll Cardiol. 2008;52(23):1834–43.
13. Kindermann M, Hennen B, Jung J, Geisel J, Bohm M, Frohlig G. Biventricular versus conventional right ventricular stimulation for patients with standard pacing indication and left ventricular dysfunction: the Homburg Biventricular Pacing Evaluation (HOBIPACE). J Am Coll Cardiol. 2006;47(10):1927–37.
14. Martinelli Filho M, de Siqueira SF, Costa R, et al. Conventional versus biventricular pacing in heart failure and bradyarrhythmia: the COMBAT study. J Card Fail. 2010;16(4):293–300.
15. Shimano M, Tsuji Y, Yoshida Y, et al. Acute and chronic effects of cardiac resynchronization in patients developing heart failure with long-term pacemaker therapy for acquired complete atrioventricular block. Europace. 2007;9(10):869–74.
16. Yu CM, Chan JY, Zhang Q, et al. Biventricular pacing in patients with bradycardia and normal ejection fraction. N Engl J Med. 2009;361(22):2123–34.
17. Chan JY, Fang F, Zhang Q, et al. Biventricular pacing is superior to right ventricular pacing in bradycardia patients with preserved systolic function: 2-year results of the PACE trial. Eur Heart J. 2011;32(20):2533–40.
18. Stockburger M, Gomez-Doblas JJ, Lamas G, et al. Preventing ventricular dysfunction in pacemaker patients without advanced heart failure: results from a multicentre international randomized trial (PREVENT-HF). Eur J Heart Fail. 2011;13(6):633–41.
19. Funck RC, Blanc JJ, Mueller HH, et al. Biventricular stimulation to prevent cardiac desynchronization: rationale, design, and endpoints of the 'Biventricular Pacing for Atrioventricular Block to Prevent Cardiac Desynchronization (BioPace)' study. Europace. 2006;8(8):629–35.
20. Funck RC, Mueller HH, Lunati M, et al. Characteristics of a large sample of candidates for permanent ventricular pacing included in the Biventricular Pacing for Atrio-ventricular Block to Prevent Cardiac Desynchronization Study (BioPace). Europace. 2014;16(3):354–62.
21. Merchant FM, Hoskins MH, Musat DL, et al. Incidence and time course for developing heart failure with high-burden right ventricular pacing. Circ Cardiovasc Qual Outcomes. 2017;10(6):1–11.
22. Doshi RN, Daoud EG, Fellows C, et al. Left ventricular-based cardiac stimulation post AV nodal ablation evaluation (the PAVE study). J Cardiovasc Electrophysiol. 2005;16(11):1160–5.
23. Curtis AB, Worley SJ, Adamson PB, et al. Biventricular pacing for atrioventricular block and systolic dysfunction. N Engl J Med. 2013;368(17):1585–93.
24. Janousek J, van Geldorp IE, Krupickova S, et al. Permanent cardiac pacing in children: choosing the optimal pacing site: a multicenter study. Circulation. 2013;127(5):613–23.
25. Motonaga KS, Dubin AM. Cardiac resynchronization therapy for pediatric patients with heart failure and congenital heart disease: a reappraisal of results. Circulation. 2014;129(18):1879–91.
26. Mittal S, Musat DL, Hoskins MH, et al. Clinical outcomes after ablation of the AV junction in 523 patients with atrial fibrillation: impact of cardiac resynchronization therapy. J Am Heart Assoc. 2017;6(12):1–12.
27. Brignole M, Botto G, Mont L, et al. Cardiac resynchronization therapy in patients undergoing atrioventricular junction ablation for permanent atrial fibrillation: a randomized trial. Eur Heart J. 2011;32(19):2420–9.
28. Nahlawi M, Waligora M, Spies SM, Bonow RO, Kadish AH, Goldberger JJ. Left ventricular function during and after right ventricular pacing. J Am Coll Cardiol. 2004;44(9):1883–8.
29. Kiehl EL, Makki T, Kumar R, et al. Incidence and predictors of right ventricular pacing-induced cardiomyopathy in patients with complete atrioventricular block and preserved left ventricular systolic function. Heart Rhythm. 2016;13(12):2272–8.
30. Prinzen FW, Peschar M. Relation between the pacing induced sequence of activation and left ventricular pump function in animals. Pacing Clin Electrophysiol. 2002;25(4 Pt 1):484–98.
31. Delhaas T, Arts T, Prinzen FW, Reneman RS. Regional fibre stress-fibre strain area as an estimate of regional blood flow and oxygen demand in the canine heart. J Physiol. 1994;477(Pt 3):481–96.

32. Lee MA, Dae MW, Langberg JJ, et al. Effects of long-term right ventricular apical pacing on left ventricular perfusion, innervation, function and histology. J Am Coll Cardiol. 1994;24(1):225–32.
33. Al-Majed NS, McAlister FA, Bakal JA, Ezekowitz JA. Meta-analysis: cardiac resynchronization therapy for patients with less symptomatic heart failure. Ann Intern Med. 2011;154(6):401–12.
34. European Heart Rhythm A, European Society of C, Heart Rhythm S, et al. 2012 EHRA/HRS expert consensus statement on cardiac resynchronization therapy in heart failure: implant and follow-up recommendations and management. Heart Rhythm. 2012;9(9):1524–76.
35. Zanon F, Ellenbogen KA, Dandamudi G, et al. Permanent his-bundle pacing: a systematic literature review and meta-analysis. Europace. 2018;20:1819–26.

Chapter 6
CRT Devices in Heart Failure: Does the Patient Need a Pacemaker or Defibrillator?

C. Normand and K. Dickstein

Introduction

Cardiac resynchronization therapy (CRT) can be delivered through CRT pacemaker devices (CRP-P) or CRTs with a defibrillator component (CRT-P). Most patients with heart failure who qualify for a CRT device also have an overlapping indication for primary prophylaxis against sudden arrhythmic death with an implantable cardioverter-defibrillator (ICD) [1, 2]. Therefore, clinicians must frequently decide whether an individual patient should receive a CRT-P or a CRT-D.

A recent survey of 11,088 patients undergoing CRT implantation conducted in Europe by the European Society of Cardiology (ESC) showed that 70% of patients were implanted with a CRT-D device and 30% with a CRT-P [3]. However, when analyzing individual countries, the percentage of CRT-P ranged from 2% to 88% [4].

International Guideline Recommendations

There is limited specific advice in international guidelines regarding the choice of device type. The ESC European Heart Rhythm Association (EHRA) guidelines suggest implanting a CRT-D in patients with a life expectancy >1 year, NYHA functional class II, ischemic heart disease, and no major comorbidities [5]. They recommend selecting a CRT-P in patients with advanced heart failure, severe renal insufficiency or dialysis, and other major comorbidities including frailty and

C. Normand · K. Dickstein (✉)
Cardiology Division, Stavanger University Hospital, Stavanger, Norway

Institute of Internal Medicine, University of Bergen, Bergen, Norway
e-mail: trout@online.no

© Springer Nature Switzerland AG 2019
J. S. Steinberg, A. E. Epstein (eds.), *Clinical Controversies in Device Therapy for Cardiac Arrhythmias*, https://doi.org/10.1007/978-3-030-22882-8_6

cachexia. The 2015 ESC guidelines for the management of patients with ventricular arrhythmias and the prevention of sudden cardiac death recommend implanting a CRT-D for prevention of sudden cardiac death (SCD) in heart failure patients in NYHA class II if their QRS is ≥130 ms, with LBBB and a LVEF ≤30% [2]. Another ESC association guideline—the Heart Failure Association (HFA)—states that, if the primary reason for implanting a CRT is to improve prognosis, most evidence lies with CRT-D for patients with NYHA functional class II and with CRT-P for patients in NYHA functional classes III to IV. If the primary reason for implanting the device is relief from symptoms, HFA guidelines propose that the clinician chooses between a CRT-P and a CRT-D, as he/she considers appropriate [1].

The Canadian Cardiac Society (CCS) guidelines suggest that a CRT-P be considered in patients who are not candidates for ICD therapy, such as those with a limited life expectancy because of significant comorbidities [6]. The NICE guidelines specific to the United Kingdom provide specific guidance on whether to implant a CRT-P or a CRT-D depending on NYHA class, QRS duration, and morphology, but do not consider the patient characteristics addressed by the EHRA guidelines [7]. The 2018 heart failure guidelines from Australia state that when CRT is indicated in most cases, a CRT-D is preferred, although, in patients with nonischemic heart failure, a CRT-P device may provide adequate protection. Furthermore, they state that—in patients who do not wish to have the potential for defibrillation, where the left ventricle is likely to improve, in the very elderly, or in those who retain a poorer prognosis but remain symptomatic—it would be reasonable to consider a CRT-P over a CRT-D [8]. American Cardiology Society recommendations relating to CRT are found in the American College of Cardiology Foundation/American Heart Association (ACCF/AHA) guidelines for the management of heart failure (2013), which were harmonized with the ACCF/AHA/Heart Rhythm Society (HRS) 2012 focused update of the 2008 guidelines for device-based therapy of cardiac rhythm abnormalities. Neither of these guidelines provide advice on choice of device type [9–11]. Furthermore, since publication of the 2013 guidelines, several focused updates of heart failure have been published by ACC/AHA/Heart Failure Society of America (HFSA). These updates do not propose changes to CRT recommendations, nor do they provide advice on choice of CRT device type [12, 13].

The Evidence for Implanting CRT-D

The recommendation for implanting a defibrillator in patients with symptomatic heart failure and reduced ejection fraction was based on the results of two large trials: the Multicenter Automatic Defibrillator Implantation Trial II (MADIT II) and the Sudden Cardiac Death in Heart Failure Trial (SCD-HeFT) [14, 15]. In MADIT II 1232 patients with prior myocardial infraction and LVEF ≤30% were randomly assigned in a 3:2 ratio to receive an ICD or optimal medical therapy (OMT). [15] In the SCD-HeFT 2521 patients with NYHA class II or II heart failure and an LVEF ≤35% were randomized to OMT, OMT and amiodarone, and OMT and ICD. Both these trials showed significantly improved survival in the patient group implanted with a defibrillator. ICDs are therefore recommended as prophylactic therapy for patients with symptomatic heart failure if their left ventricular ejection fraction is ≤35% [2]. A logical extrapolation would therefore be that in the patient group with a wide QRS qualifying for CRT, the preferred choice would be a CRT-D.

The Evidence for Implanting a CRT-P vs. a CRT-D

The Evidence for CRT-P Alone

One of the pivotal CRT trials, CARE HF, randomized 813 patients to OMT with or without CRT. This trial convincingly demonstrated a reduction in total mortality with CRT compared with optimal medical therapy in eligible patients [16]. In the extended follow-up dataset, CRT-P was associated with a reduction in sudden cardiac death closely correlated to LV reverse remodeling [17, 18]. In addition, the REVERSE study that randomized 610 patients with mild heart failure to active or inactive CRT therapy demonstrated that significant reverse LV remodeling was associated with a reduction in ventricular tachycardia (VT). [19]. Furthermore, in the MADIT-CRT trial where 1820 patients with EF ≤30% and QRS >130 ms with mild heart failure were randomized to CRT-D or ICD, reverse remodeling was also associated with a significant reduction in the risk of subsequent life-threatening VT [20].

Therefore, the question remains: Does the addition of a defibrillator offer additional protection to these patients receiving a CRT device? Furthermore, if CRT-D patients need their device replaced, should they perhaps receive a CRT-P instead? This is an important question to answer, as the addition of the defibrillator component is not without potential adverse procedural complications including the risk of inappropriate shocks [21, 22]. In the follow-up analysis of the MADIT II trial (ICD vs. OMT) [15], the investigators found that 11.5% of the 719 patients receiving an ICD experienced an inappropriate shock [21]. The most common trigger for these shocks was atrial fibrillation. Noteworthily, these patients had higher mortality rates than those who did not receive inappropriate shocks (hazard ratio 2.29, $p = 0.025$). Another retrospective cohort study compared inappropriate shocks in 85 patients implanted with a CRT-D with 100 patients implanted with an ICD device with a follow-up period of 21 ± 13 months [23]. In this study 18 patients experienced inappropriate shocks. However, there was significantly lower rate of inappropriate shock in the CRT-D group vs. the ICD group. Again, atrial fibrillation and atrial flutter were the strongest predictors of inappropriate shocks. The authors therefore suggest that CRT, by reducing the atrial fibrillation burden in these patients, is responsible for lower rate of inappropriate shocks compared with the ICD patients.

One might also assume that implanting an ICD lead with its increased size and rigidity would lead to more periprocedural complications than implanting only the right and left ventricular CRT pacing leads. However, the evidence is conflicting. A 2013 Danish cohort study of 5918 patients with cardiac implantable electronic devices found that implantation of a CRT-D compared with a CRT-P was associated with a higher risk of complications, primarily due to lead-related re-interventions (CRT-D 4.7 vs. 2.3% CRT-P, $P = 0.001$) [22]. Another study looking at 1-year outcomes of 402 CRT-P and CRT-D implantations found that CRT-D patients had higher incidences of loss of capture (CRT-D 9.2% vs. 3.5% CRT-P, $P = 0.01$). However, in this study there were no significant differences in infections rates, rehospitalization rates, and mortality rates between the two groups [24]. Furthermore, the ESC CRT Survey II (11,088 patients) and a recent multicenter European cohort study (3008 patients) with CRT-P and CRT-D implantations found similar periprocedural complication rates between both CRT-P and CRT-D recipients [4, 25]. The CRT Survey II also reported similar adverse event rates during hospitalization and similar length of stay between the two groups [4]. This could reflect increased international implantation experience or possibly a choice for CRT-P in patients deemed at higher risk for complications. Although the periprocedural complications were the same in the European cohort study of 3008 patients, they did find significant differences between the groups in late complications in this study during a mean follow-up of 41.4 ± 29 months. The significantly higher rate of complications in the CRT-D group was particularly evident for device-related infections [25].

In addition, one must remember that in a substantial portion of patients who receive a CRT-D or ICD, the device never fires [26]. Furthermore, the defibrillator device has a higher cost than a device with only a pacemaker component and requires a more intensive follow-up program [27].

Direct Comparisons of CRT- P vs. CRT-D

No adequately powered, randomized clinical trial has compared the effect of CRT-P vs. CRT-D on long-term clinical outcomes in eligible patients. Only one head-to-head study of CRT-D vs. CRT-P has ever been published. However, this study (COMPANION) with 1520 patients was not designed to compare different CRT devices; rather, it focused on the overall concept of CRT versus optimal medical therapy. The study had three arms: OMT alone, OMT + CRT-P, or OMT with CRT-D. It established the benefit of a CRT over medical therapy in eligible patients, but was underpowered to compare any difference between the two device arms. Although total mortality was only reduced compared with medical therapy in the CRT-D arm, the CRT-P and CRT-D curves largely overlapped one another [28].

The majority of comparisons of CRT-P vs. CRT-D have been retrospective cohort studies, and these have suggested that the benefit for a CRT-D over a CRT-P may be limited to those patients with ischemic heart failure etiology. A study from a high-volume single center, comparing the mortality rates of 693 patients implanted with a CRT-P vs. 429 implanted with a CRT-D, found CRT-D to be associated with a 30% risk reduction in all-cause mortality compared with a CRT-P. However, such a mortality benefit was not observed for patients with nonischemic cardiomyopathy [27]. Another observational study of 5307 consecutive patients with CRT-P vs. CRT-D again only found improved survival in the patients with ischemic heart failure with a CRT-D. In the patients with nonischemic heart failure there was no mortality benefit from a CRT-D vs. a CRT-P [29]. In a UK cohort study of 551 patients implanted with a CRT-D versus 999 with a CRT-P, CRT-D was associated with lower mortality, heart failure hospitalizations, and hospitalizations for major acute coronary events (MACE) after stratifying for heart failure etiology; this lower mortality rate was only evident for the patients with ischemic heart failure etiology [30].

The only recent RCT of defibrillator over standard care, the DANISH study, randomized 556 patients with heart failure of nonischemic etiology with an LVEF ≤35% to either receive an ICD or usual clinical care. Despite the rate of sudden cardiac death being half in the ICD group (4.3%) compared with the control group (8.2%), this trial showed no significant difference in overall survival benefit between the two groups. There was, however, an age interaction suggesting that the benefits of ICD in patients with nonischemic etiology were limited to the younger patients (<68 years of age) [31]. In both the ICD and the control group 58% of the patients received a CRT device, and these results were independent of whether or not the patients received a CRT. Therefore, this study enabled the direct comparison of 323 CRT-P patients versus 322 CRT-D patients with ischemic heart failure etiology. The DANISH study suggests that in patients >68 years of age with heart failure due to nonischemic etiology, the increased mortality rate is not due to sudden cardiac death but rather to another mode of death for which an ICD does not improve mortality rates.

This futility of the defibrillator in patients ≥75 years of age is further supported by a study examining 775 consecutive patients undergoing CRT implantations [32]. Of the 177 patients that fulfilled the inclusion criteria, 80 were implanted with a CRT-P and 97 with a CRT-D. After 26 ± 19 months, 35% of patients had died with no significant difference between the two groups, 35% in the CRT-P and 35% in the CRT-D group ($p = 0.994$).

In the French CeRtiTuDe registry, 1705 recipients of either a CRT-P or a CRT-D were followed rigorously for adjudicated causes of death over 2 years [33]. Patients with CRT-P compared with CRT-D were older (mean age 76 years), were less often male, had more symptoms of heart failure, and less often had ischemic etiology, and more patients had atrial fibrillation and other comorbidities. Although in CeRtiTuDe mortality was double in the CRT-P vs. the CRT-D group, this increased mortality rate was due to non-sudden cardiac death in the CRT-P group, thereby suggesting that the patients that are routinely selected for a CRT-P would not benefit from a CRT-D.

A large single-center study published in 2016 showed results similar to the CeRtiTuDe registry, namely, that despite being younger and fitter, recipients of CRT-D systems did not have a clear mortality benefit over those that received CRT-P systems [34]. In short, CRT reduces but probably does not completely abolish the risk of sudden cardiac death. The likely mechanism is related to reverse remodeling following successful resynchronization [20].

Which Patients Are Getting Which Device Type?

The percentage of CRT-P vs. CRT-D varies greatly in different regions and countries as shown in Figs. 6.1 and 6.2 [4, 35]. In Europe the percentage of CRT-P devices ranged from as low as 2% to as high as 88%. The variation could not be explained simply by the country's economic status, so clearly other factors are motivating physicians to make choices between CRT-P and CRT-D. In a cross-sectional study from the United States, looking at 311,086 CRT implantations, they found that 86.1% were CRT-Ds [36].

In the CRT Survey II, the CRT-P recipients were older, more commonly had NYHA functional class III–IV symptoms, were more often female, had higher NT-pro BNP levels, and more frequently had comorbidities and additional conduction tissue disease. On the other hand, patients implanted with a CRT-D device were more likely to have ischemic heart failure etiology. A large meta-analysis in patients with CRT-P vs. CRT-D comprising 44 studies and 18,874 patients found that CRT-P recipients were older, were more often female, and had higher NYHA class, with more atrial fibrillation and less ischemic heart disease. This study found an unadjusted mortality rate that was twofold higher in the patients with CRT-P with SCD representing a third of the excess mortality [37], thereby suggesting that patients with higher NYHA class and more comorbidities are being selected for CRT-P over CRT-D.

Furthermore, an analysis of data from patients >75 years of age evaluated 405 patients with a CRT-D and 107 patients with a CRT-P and found that the increased mortality of the CRT-P groups was lost when adjusting for the baseline differences

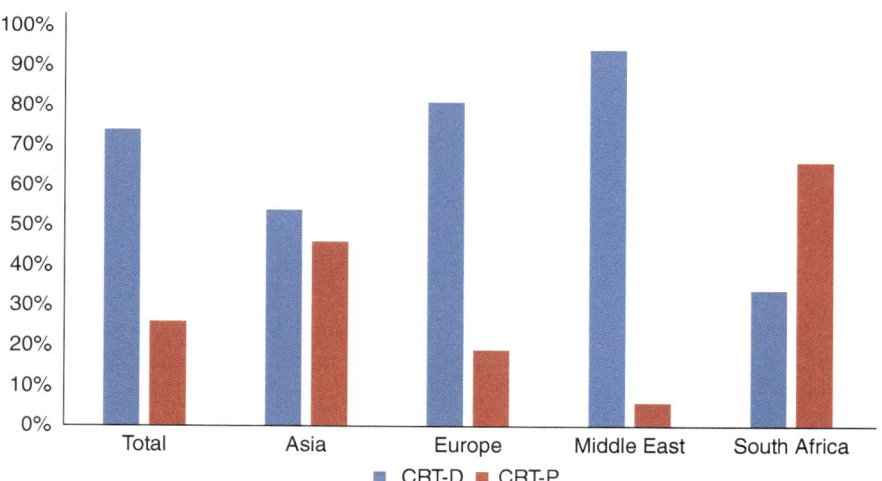

Fig. 6.1 CRT-P vs. CRT-D in different regions. (Adapted from Bastian D, Ebrahim IO, Chen JY et al. Real-world geographic variations in the use of cardiac implantable electronic devices-The PANORAMA 2 observational cohort study. Pacing and clinical electrophysiology: PACE 2018)

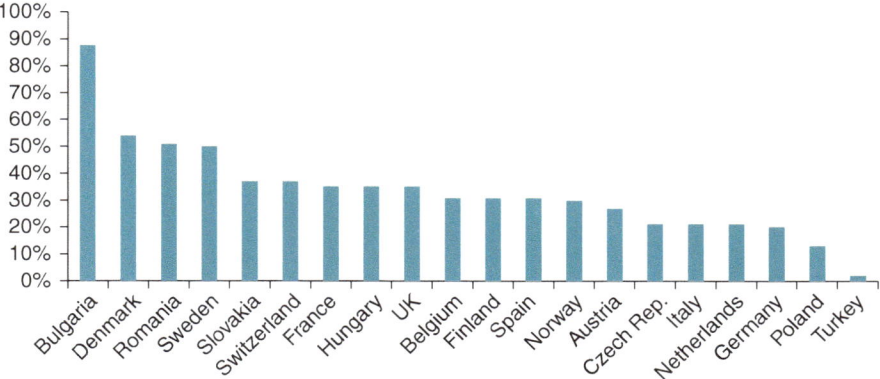

Fig. 6.2 Percentage CRT-P per country in Europe

between the groups. These variables included age (the CRT-P groups were older (83 years vs. 81 years, $P < 0.001$)) and more extensive comorbidities (Charlson index = 5 [3–6] vs. 4 [3–5], $P = 0.007$) [38].

How Should We Proceed?

Perhaps providing implanters with a scoring system for patient selection would assist in appropriate patient selection. A risk score called the Goldenberg risk score has been proposed to identify patients with a limited survival benefit from a CRT-D, who may therefore be implanted with a CRT-P rather than a CRT-D. This risk score includes five clinical risk factors including NYHA class >2, atrial fibrillation, QRS duration >120 ms, age >70 years, and blood urea nitrogen >26 mg/dl. In a retrospective observational cohort study of 638 patients, it was found that patients with a low score of 0–2 had a decreased mortality rate compared with a CRT-P in the first 4 years of follow-up (CRT-D 11.3 vs. CRT-P 24.7%, $P = 0.041$). Although this effect attenuated with longer follow-up duration (CRT-D 21.2 vs. CRT-P 32.7%, $P = 0.078$), no significant benefit of a CRT-D was found in those with a risk score ≥3. Such risk scores may prove useful in informing the selection of the most appropriate type of CRT device in the individual patient [39].

However, in order to properly resolve the P vs. D question, we would require a large, randomized controlled trial directly comparing the two types of CRT devices on long-term clinical outcomes. Such an ambitious trial would necessarily have to include sufficient numbers of patients to permit evaluation of the outcomes in the various clinical subgroups. Fortunately, the RESET-CRT trial is underway in Germany (ClinicalTrials.gov number NCT03494933). In this study, 2030 patients with both ischemic and nonischemic HF etiology will be randomized to a CRT-P or CRT-D with the following inclusion criteria: >18 years of age, symptomatic heart failure (NYHA class II–IV), LVEF ≤35%, on OMT, and with a class I or IIa indication for a CRT device. Patients with a previous VT episode and those with a I or IIa indication for secondary prevention of sudden cardiac death and VT with an ICD are excluded. The primary endpoint of this study is all-cause mortality. Hopefully, the results of such a trial will shed more light on this important and clinically relevant issue.

Conclusion

Faced with many competing causes of death in patients with heart failure and left ventricular dysfunction, the selection of patients who might benefit from a CRT-D is challenging. We should estimate clinically whether the patient is expected to survive at least 1 year with good functional status before implanting a CRT-D. Furthermore, the likelihood of sudden cardiac death should be evaluated and outweigh the potential adverse events associated with the device. However, a CRT-P might also provide adequate protection from the increased mortality risk that these patients face, and they might not require the defibrillator component. This important question can only be adequately addressed by a large RCT comparing both devices in sufficient subgroups of eligible patients with heart failure and left ventricular systolic dysfunction.

References

1. Ponikowski P, Voors AA, Anker SD, et al. 2016 ESC guidelines for the diagnosis and treatment of acute and chronic heart failure: the Task Force for the diagnosis and treatment of acute and chronic heart failure of the European Society of Cardiology (ESC). Developed with the special contribution of the Heart Failure Association (HFA) of the ESC. Eur J Heart Fail. 2016;18:891–975.
2. Authors/Task Force M, Priori SG, Blomstrom-Lundqvist C, et al. 2015 ESC guidelines for the management of patients with ventricular arrhythmias and the prevention of sudden cardiac death: the Task Force for the Management of Patients with Ventricular Arrhythmias and the Prevention of Sudden Cardiac Death of the European Society of Cardiology (ESC)Endorsed by: Association for European Paediatric and Congenital Cardiology (AEPC). Europace. 2015;17:1601–87.
3. Dickstein K, Normand C, Auricchio A, et al. CRT survey II: a European Society of Cardiology survey of cardiac resynchronisation therapy in 11 088 patients-who is doing what to whom and how? Eur J Heart Fail. 2018;20(6):1039–51.
4. Normand CLC, Bogale N, et al. Cardiac resynchronization therapy pacemaker or cardiac resynchronization therapy defibrillator: what determines the choice?—findings from the ESC CRT survey II. Europace. 2019;21(6):918–27.
5. Brignole M, Auricchio A, Baron-Esquivias G, et al. 2013 ESC guidelines on cardiac pacing and cardiac resynchronization therapy: the Task Force on cardiac pacing and resynchronization therapy of the European Society of Cardiology (ESC). Developed in collaboration with the European Heart Rhythm Association (EHRA). Eur Heart J. 2013;34:2281–329.

6. Ezekowitz JA, O'Meara E, McDonald MA, et al. 2017 Comprehensive update of the Canadian Cardiovascular Society Guidelines for the Management of Heart Failure. Can J Cardiol. 2017;33:1342–433.
7. NICE. Implantable cardioverter defibrillators and cardiac resynchronisation therapy for arrhythmias and heart failure (review of TA95 and TA120). guidance.nice.org.uk/ta314: NICE, 2014.
8. Group NCHFGW, Atherton JJ, Sindone A, et al. National Heart Foundation of Australia and Cardiac Society of Australia and New Zealand: guidelines for the prevention, detection, and management of heart failure in Australia 2018. Heart Lung Circ. 2018;27:1123–208.
9. Normand C, Linde C, Singh J, Dickstein K. Indications for cardiac resynchronization therapy: a comparison of the major international guidelines. JACC Heart Fail. 2018;6:308–16.
10. Yancy CW, Jessup M, Bozkurt B, et al. 2013 ACCF/AHA guideline for the management of heart failure: executive summary: a report of the American College of Cardiology Foundation/American Heart Association Task Force on practice guidelines. Circulation. 2013;128:1810–52.
11. Tracy CM, Epstein AE, Darbar D, et al. 2012 ACCF/AHA/HRS focused update of the 2008 guidelines for device-based therapy of cardiac rhythm abnormalities: a report of the American College of Cardiology Foundation/American Heart Association Task Force on practice guidelines and the Heart Rhythm Society. [corrected]. Circulation. 2012;126:1784–800.
12. Yancy CW, Jessup M, Bozkurt B, et al. 2016 ACC/AHA/HFSA focused update on new pharmacological therapy for heart failure: an update of the 2013 ACCF/AHA guideline for the management of heart failure: a report of the American College of Cardiology/American Heart Association Task Force on Clinical Practice Guidelines and the Heart Failure Society of America. J Am Coll Cardiol. 2016;68:1476–88.
13. Yancy CW, Jessup M, Bozkurt B, et al. 2017 ACC/AHA/HFSA focused update of the 2013 ACCF/AHA guideline for the management of heart failure: a report of the American College of Cardiology/American Heart Association Task Force on Clinical Practice Guidelines and the Heart Failure Society of America. J Card Fail. 2017;23:628–51.
14. Bardy GH, Lee KL, Mark DB, et al. Amiodarone or an implantable cardioverter-defibrillator for congestive heart failure. N Engl J Med. 2005;352:225–37.
15. Moss AJ, Zareba W, Hall WJ, et al. Prophylactic implantation of a defibrillator in patients with myocardial infarction and reduced ejection fraction. N Engl J Med. 2002;346:877–83.
16. Cleland JG, Daubert JC, Erdmann E, et al. The effect of cardiac resynchronization on morbidity and mortality in heart failure. N Engl J Med. 2005;352:1539–49.
17. Ghio S, Freemantle N, Scelsi L, et al. Long-term left ventricular reverse remodelling with cardiac resynchronization therapy: results from the CARE-HF trial. Eur J Heart Fail. 2009;11:480–8.
18. Cleland JG, Daubert JC, Erdmann E, et al. Longer-term effects of cardiac resynchronization therapy on mortality in heart failure [the CArdiac REsynchronization-Heart Failure (CARE-HF) trial extension phase]. Eur Heart J. 2006;27:1928–32.
19. Gold MR, Linde C, Abraham WT, Gardiwal A, Daubert JC. The impact of cardiac resynchronization therapy on the incidence of ventricular arrhythmias in mild heart failure. Heart Rhythm. 2011;8:679–84.
20. Barsheshet A, Wang PJ, Moss AJ, et al. Reverse remodeling and the risk of ventricular tachyarrhythmias in the MADIT-CRT (Multicenter Automatic Defibrillator Implantation Trial-Cardiac Resynchronization Therapy). J Am Coll Cardiol. 2011;57:2416–23.
21. Daubert JP, Zareba W, Cannom DS, et al. Inappropriate implantable cardioverter-defibrillator shocks in MADIT II: frequency, mechanisms, predictors, and survival impact. J Am Coll Cardiol. 2008;51:1357–65.
22. Kirkfeldt RE, Johansen JB, Nohr EA, Jorgensen OD, Nielsen JC. Complications after cardiac implantable electronic device implantations: an analysis of a complete, nationwide cohort in Denmark. Eur Heart J. 2014;35:1186–94.
23. Chen Z, Kotecha T, Crichton S, et al. Lower incidence of inappropriate shock therapy in patients with combined cardiac resynchronisation therapy defibrillators (CRT-D) compared with patients with non-CRT defibrillators (ICDs). Int J Clin Pract. 2013;67:733–9.

24. Schuchert A, Muto C, Maounis T, et al. Lead complications, device infections, and clinical outcomes in the first year after implantation of cardiac resynchronization therapy-defibrillator and cardiac resynchronization therapy-pacemaker. Europace. 2013;15:71–6.
25. Barra S, Providencia R, Boveda S, et al. Device complications with addition of defibrillation to cardiac resynchronisation therapy for primary prevention. Heart. 2018;104:1529–35.
26. Stevenson LW, Desai AS. Selecting patients for discussion of the ICD as primary prevention for sudden death in heart failure. J Card Fail. 2006;12:407–12.
27. Kutyifa V, Geller L, Bogyi P, et al. Effect of cardiac resynchronization therapy with implantable cardioverter defibrillator versus cardiac resynchronization therapy with pacemaker on mortality in heart failure patients: results of a high-volume, single-centre experience. Eur J Heart Fail. 2014;16:1323–30.
28. Bristow MR, Saxon LA, Boehmer J, et al. Cardiac-resynchronization therapy with or without an implantable defibrillator in advanced chronic heart failure. N Engl J Med. 2004;350:2140–50.
29. Barra S, Boveda S, Providencia R, et al. Adding defibrillation therapy to cardiac resynchronization on the basis of the myocardial substrate. J Am Coll Cardiol. 2017;69:1669–78.
30. Leyva F, Zegard A, Umar F, et al. Long-term clinical outcomes of cardiac resynchronization therapy with or without defibrillation: impact of the aetiology of cardiomyopathy. Europace. 2018;20:1804–12.
31. Kober L, Thune JJ, Nielsen JC, et al. Defibrillator implantation in patients with nonischemic systolic heart failure. N Engl J Med. 2016;375:1221–30.
32. Doring M, Ebert M, Dagres N, et al. Cardiac resynchronization therapy in the ageing population – with or without an implantable defibrillator? Int J Cardiol. 2018;263:48–53.
33. Marijon E, Leclercq C, Narayanan K, et al. Causes-of-death analysis of patients with cardiac resynchronization therapy: an analysis of the CeRtiTuDe cohort study. Eur Heart J. 2015;36:2767–76.
34. Drozd M, Gierula J, Lowry JE, et al. Cardiac resynchronization therapy outcomes in patients with chronic heart failure: cardiac resynchronization therapy with pacemaker versus cardiac resynchronization therapy with defibrillator. J Cardiovasc Med. 2017;18:962–7.
35. Bastian D, Ebrahim IO, Chen JY et al. Real-world geographic variations in the use of cardiac implantable electronic devices-The PANORAMA 2 observational cohort study. Pacing Clin Electrophysiol (PACE). 2018;41(8):978–89.
36. Lindvall C, Chatterjee NA, Chang Y, et al. National trends in the use of cardiac resynchronization therapy with or without implantable cardioverter-defibrillator. Circulation. 2016;133:273–81.
37. Barra S, Providencia R, Duehmke R, et al. Cause-of-death analysis in patients with cardiac resynchronization therapy with or without a defibrillator: a systematic review and proportional meta-analysis. Europace. 2018;20:481–91.
38. Munir MB, Althouse AD, Rijal S, et al. Clinical characteristics and outcomes of older cardiac resynchronization therapy recipients using a pacemaker versus a defibrillator. J Cardiovasc Electrophysiol. 2016;27:730–4.
39. Barra S, Looi KL, Gajendragadkar PR, Khan FZ, Virdee M, Agarwal S. Applicability of a risk score for prediction of the long-term benefit of the implantable cardioverter defibrillator in patients receiving cardiac resynchronization therapy. Europace. 2016;18:1187–93.

Chapter 7
His Bundle Pacing Versus Biventricular Pacing for CRT

Nicole Habel and Daniel L. Lustgarten

Cardiac resynchronization therapy (CRT) by the way of biventricular (BiV) pacing is an established component of heart failure treatment in selected patients[1] and aims at reestablishing synchrony between right ventricular and left ventricular activation [1]. However, this form of cardiac excitation fails to emulate the multisite simultaneous endo- to epicardial activation resulting in torsional contraction, which is critical to achieve optimal cardiac output.

His bundle pacing (HBP) offers an alternative to biventricular pacing by engaging intact His-Purkinje fibers, thereby restoring physiologic ventricular activation. Contrary to common belief, the anatomic location of the bundle of His makes it amendable to pacing in the majority of patients, and procedural techniques have become less challenging since the availability of sheath delivery systems.

Evolution of Pacing

The evolution of pacing began with a focus on working with the constraints of technology, with little emphasis on interacting with the anatomy of the native conduction system. The first electronic pacemaker was enormous due to the absence of transistors, the advent of which permitted the development of smaller batteries, the first ones being externalized devices that were soon followed by implantable ones. Further miniaturization and more sophisticated leads brought us to the current paradigm. Cardiac resynchronization therapy mirrors the history of the implantable pacemaker, with the focus being placed on further engineering improvements

---

[1] CRT is indicated in systolic heart failure NYHA class II–IV, with LVEF $\leq 35\%$ and LBBB with QRS ≥ 150 ms (class I recommendation – 2012 focused update of 2008 guidelines).

N. Habel · D. L. Lustgarten (✉)
University of Vermont Medical Center, Burlington, VT, USA
e-mail: Nicole.Habel@uvmhealth.org; Daniel.Lustgarten@uvmhealth.org

© Springer Nature Switzerland AG 2019   87
J. S. Steinberg, A. E. Epstein (eds.), *Clinical Controversies in Device Therapy for Cardiac Arrhythmias*, https://doi.org/10.1007/978-3-030-22882-8_7

and – up until recently – relatively little attention to understanding the relationship between pacing sites and the specialized conduction system.

The detrimental effect of interventricular asynchrony was already recognized by Wiggers in 1925 when examining the maximum LV pressure derivative (LV dP/dt max) of canine myocardium in response to surface stimulation [2]. Once radionuclide ventriculography became available in the 1980s, Grines et al. [3] described significantly lower LVEF in 18 patients with left bundle branch block (LBBB) as compared to 10 normal subjects and de Teresa showed reversal of this effect when pacing the LV free wall [4]. Biventricular pacing in heart failure was first implemented in 1993: Bakker and colleagues [5] treated 12 patients with advanced heart failure, sinus rhythm, and LBBB with biventricular stimulation by implanting a dual-chamber pacemaker and affixing an epicardial lead to the anterolateral LV wall via minithoracotomy. Functional capacity improved from median NYHA class IV to II–III in the short term and was sustained at 1-year follow-up in those patients who survived to 12 months (9/12 patients). Transvenous LV lead insertion was tested in the mid-1990s [6] and paved the way for systematic evaluation of BiV pacing for CRT.

The Multisite Stimulation in Cardiomyopathy (MUSTIC) trial [7], published in 2001, was the first randomized controlled trial to show clinical benefit from CRT by means of biventricular pacing. While MUSTIC and MIRACLE [8] showed improvements in symptoms and functional parameters, the 2004 COMPANION trial [9] suggested biventricular pacing – even in the absence of defibrillation – conveys a mortality benefit. Subsequent studies provided further evidence for BiV pacing reducing the composite primary endpoint of heart failure hospitalization and all-cause mortality when compared to medical therapy alone (CARE-HF [10]) or defibrillator implant alone (MADIT-CRT [11]). Unfortunately, the rate of nonresponders (i.e., failure to improve mortality, LV function, or symptoms) ranges between 20% and 40%. This has stimulated research into technical improvements, optimizing patient selection as well as, LV lead and site selection. Subgroup analysis of MADIT-CRT [12] and REVERSE [13] showed no benefit in patients with non-LBBB morphology, and a 2012 meta-analysis suggested lack of benefit from CRT in patient with QRS duration <150 ms [14]. LV lead positioning is anatomically ideal in the lateral or posterolateral aspect of the LV wall; however this can be limited by variations in coronary sinus branch vessels and fails to account for individual electrical/mechanical delay. Additionally, inadvertent phrenic nerve stimulation by traditional bipolar LV leads can be clinically relevant in up to 22% of patients [15]. Quadripolar pacing leads and leadless LV pacing are technical solutions developed or being developed in an attempt to circumnavigate these issues, but neither addresses the fact that ventricular myocyte pacing is non-physiologic. His bundle pacing on the other hand offers a physiologic approach to resynchronization by addressing the underlying issue of abnormal conduction.

Anatomy and Physiology of the His Bundle

In the absence of conduction disturbance within the His-Purkinje system, earliest ventricular activation usually occurs at the left ventricular side of the mid-septum.

Excitation then spreads across the septum from left to right and from the apex toward the base, with the posterobasal area of the left ventricle usually being activated last [16]. This pattern of ventricular activation is critical toward generating optimal torsional and compressive ventricular contraction. Even though biventricular pacing can engage myocardial segments in simultaneous contraction, it fails to restore longitudinal shortening of the septum, which is crucial to the ventricular twisting motion [17]. Hence, pacing the His bundle with re-engagement of latent fascicular tissue can potentiate reestablishment of optimal electromechanical coupling.

Anatomic and histologic studies by Tawara and colleagues [18, 19] in the early twentieth century provide the foundation for our understanding of the specialized conduction system of the heart. The bundle of His is a direct continuation of the AV node and penetrates the central fibrous body at the apex of the triangle of Koch. It continues undivided for approximately 11 mm (range 7–15 mm) [20] before the separation into anterior left bundle branch (LBB), posterior LBB, and right bundle branch (RBB) [21]. A recent study by Kawashima [22] elegantly demonstrates the topological relationship of the His bundle to the membranous part of the intraventricular septum and its depth from the endocardium. They found three types of variation, with a superficial location of the His bundle in the majority of cases (68%, types I and III):

- Type I: 49/105 cases (Fig. 7.1a) – The His bundle is located under a thin layer of myocytes at the lower border of the membranous part of the interventricular septum.

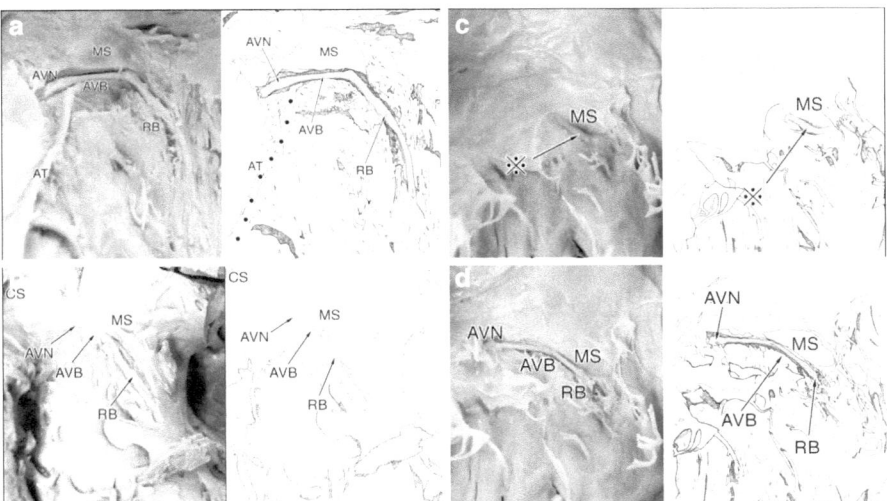

Fig. 7.1 Adopted from Kawashima et al. [22]. Anatomic relationship of the atrioventricular bundle to the membranous septum. (**a**) Thin layer of myocardium covers the bundle of His (46.7%). (**b**) The His bundle runs within the interventricular muscle (32.4%). (**c**) "Naked" His bundle – Asterisk denotes exposed His bundle prior to dissection. (**d**) "Naked" His bundle after dissection (21.0%)

Fig. 7.2 Schematic
of longitudinal separation
of Purkinje strands.
TA tricuspid annulus

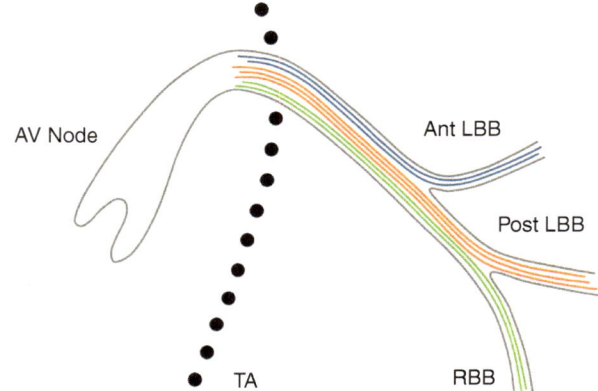

- Type II: 34/105 cases (Fig. 7.1b) – The His bundle runs within the interventricular muscle.
- Type III: 22/105 cases (Fig. 7.1c, d) – The His bundle was located immediately underneath the endocardium coursing directly across the membranous part of the interventricular septum ("naked His bundle").

Ultrastructural examination of the bundle of His by James and Sherf [23] demonstrated collagen-mediated longitudinal separation of Purkinje strands with gap junctions predominantly distributed end-to-end with less intercellular coupling present transversely. This discovery leads to the hypothesis that the His bundle is not just a loose interconnected conglomerate of Purkinje fibers that eventually separates into the trifascicular conduction system, but rather that the individual bundle branches are functionally defined within the His bundle (Fig. 7.2).

Accordingly, on the bases of these anatomical observations, it was expected that bundle branch block might be a manifestation of disease in the His bundle, the latter causing longitudinal dissociation with favored conduction down one fascicle or bundle relative to another. This model was supported by findings like those of Onkar Narula, who in 1977 [24] published a report in which he demonstrated normalization of the QRS in 25 out of 80 patients studied who had left bundle branch block. Furthermore, he noted that pacing the His bundle slightly more proximal to the site demonstrating normalization resulted in the baseline conduction defect, thereby supporting the longitudinal dissociation hypothesis.

His Bundle Pacing

Scherlag and colleagues [25] were the first to demonstrate that physiologic ventricular activation can be achieved by inserting fine Teflon-coated stainless steel wires into the proximal His bundle located within the atrioventricular septum in an in vivo canine model. In 1970 Narula [26] succeeded in transvenously pacing the

His bundle in humans and only a few years later reported on the differential effect of proximal vs. distal His bundle pacing in patient with left bundle branch block.

Engaging the bundle of His through pacing can manifest in two ways: (1) Selective His bundle capture refers to the sole recruitment of His-Purkinje fibers resulting in identical paced and intrinsic QRS morphology, QRS, and T-wave concordance as well as similar Stim-V and H-V interval.[2] (2) Nonselective His bundle capture on the other hand represents the fusion of His-Purkinje and adjacent local ventricular activation resulting in short Stim-V interval and altered QRS morphology depending on output.

In 2000 Deshmukh et al. [27] described the first experience of permanent His bundle pacing in patients with chronic atrial fibrillation, dilated cardiomyopathy with LVEF <40%, NYHA class III–IV, and normal QRS width. The authors were able to actively fix a standard pacing lead at the atrioventricular septum in 12 out of 18 patients. The lead (with the screw exposed and the aid of a hand-modified J-shaped stylet) was positioned near a hexapolar His mapping catheter and maneuvered to obtain the largest His potential possible. This initial study provided promising results: LVEF improved significantly from $18.2 \pm 9.8\%$ to $28.6 \pm 11.2\%$ ($p < 0.05$) over 8–35 months of follow-up and 9 out of 11 patients had improved NYHA functional class. A follow-up study in 2004 [28] with 39/54 patients successfully undergoing HBP demonstrated improved LVEF as well as increased cardiopulmonary exercise capacity.

Stable positioning of the lead within the atrioventricular septum was challenging during the early experience using a 1.5 mm helical screw and a J-shaped stylet [27]; however in 2006 Zanon [29] reported a 92% success rate using a delivery system that includes a steerable sheath and a longer 1.8 mm helical screw. More recently, Sharma and colleagues [30] achieved HBP in 80% of patients utilizing a fixed-shaped double-curved sheath along with a 1.8 mm helical screw, but without an additional His mapping catheter. The His bundle can be approached on either the atrial or ventricular side of the tricuspid valve, as illustrated in Fig. 7.3. An autopsy report by Correa da Sa [31] provides macroscopic and microscopic evidence that the His bundle can be accessed from the atrial side of the tricuspid annulus (Fig. 7.4). A stepwise approach to implanting His bundle leads has been described elsewhere [32]. In spite of early concerns of lead failure with the His bundle pacing lead, stability has proven to be comparable to LV leads in terms of stability and threshold changes [29, 33, 34] and has been shown to exhibit similar dislodgment rates to RV pacing, albeit in centers with extensive experience with the procedure [30].

His bundle pacing as an alternative to biventricular pacing to implement resynchronization in CRT-indicated patients was initially studied by Lustgarten et al. [35], who demonstrated that eight out of ten consecutive patients acutely normalized their QRS in response to a temporarily actively fixed pacing lead, suggesting that His-CRT could be feasible. Subsequently, a direct crossover comparison of BiV and His bundle pacing was published [36] to explore whether or not a clinical response could be demonstrated. After a 6-month follow-up with each pacing modality, similar improvements with BiV and His bundle pacing were noted with a

---

[2] Selective His bundle capture is only identical to intrinsic conduction if bundle branch disease is absent at baseline. Underlying bundle branch block can normalize with His bundle pacing.

Fig. 7.3 Schematic of atrial and ventricular approach to His bundle pacing

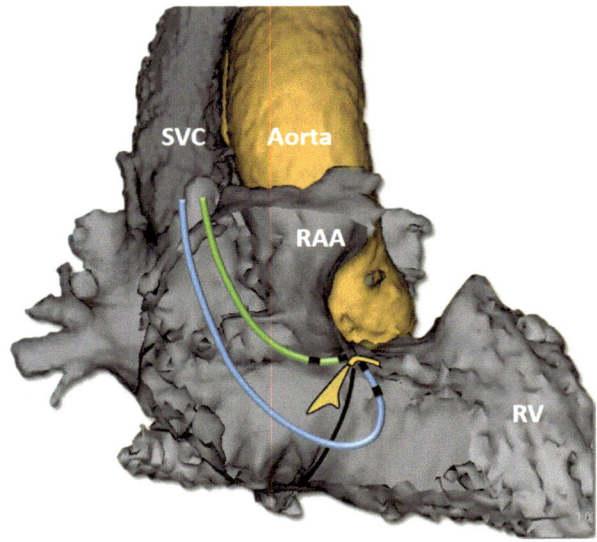

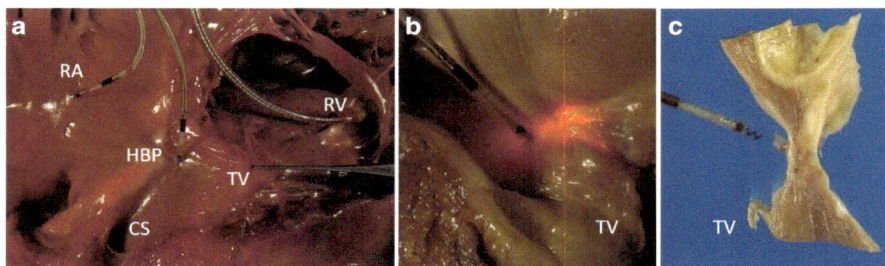

Fig. 7.4 Adopted from Correa de Sa et al. [31]. (**a**) His bundle pacing lead is implanted on the atrial side of the tricuspid annulus. (**b**) Transillumination of the membranous septum following formalin fixation, showing location of the His bundle lead at the superior aspect of the membranous septum. (**c**) His bundle lead insertion site 9 mm above the tricuspid valve leaflet

trend toward improved EF, quality of life, 6-min walk test, and a significant improvement in NYHA functional class (2.9 at baseline and 1.9 for both HBP and BiV pacing). Since this report there have been prospective observational studies of His-CRT demonstrating clinical responses with higher proportions of super-response relative to previously published BiV-CRT studies. Prospective randomized comparisons are now needed to examine outcome differences between these two modalities, but with current published series, it is reasonable to consider His bundle pacing for BiV nonresponders or patients in whom LV lead placement failed (as illustrated in the cases below). Based on recent data from Sharma and colleagues [37], His bundle pacing should also be considered in patients with heart failure and RBBB – in a series of 39 patients, HBP had a positive effect on LVEF (increase from $31 \pm 10\%$ to $39 \pm 13\%$, $p = 0.004$) along with improvement in NYHA functional class.

The following cases are examples of CRT-indicated patients in whom for different reasons biventricular pacing failed as a treatment option:

Case I

A 59-year-old male with ischemic cardiomyopathy and left bundle branch block, who recently underwent coronary artery bypass grafting, had persistently reduced LVEF of 25–30% at the 4-month postsurgical follow-up and hence was referred for CRT-D. LV lead placement was attempted via the coronary sinus. The patient had a single lateral vein, which was tortuous and acutely angled, and multiple cannulation attempts failed. An octapolar mapping catheter was advanced via a separate axillary sheath and pacing at a mapped His site normalized the QRS pattern intermittently. A His lead was implanted adjacent to the bipolar electrode pair on the mapping catheter where the His electrogram was being visualized. His capture (Fig. 7.5) re-engages the left bundle (note QRS morphology change) and results in significant shortening of "Stim to end of QRS" (first beat) as compared to "His to end of QRS" with native conduction (second beat), and as can be noted on the second beat, a His potential demonstrating injury current is evident on the His bundle pacing lead. The patient's LVEF immediately increased to 40% post-procedurally and further improved to 45–50% at 5 months of follow-up.

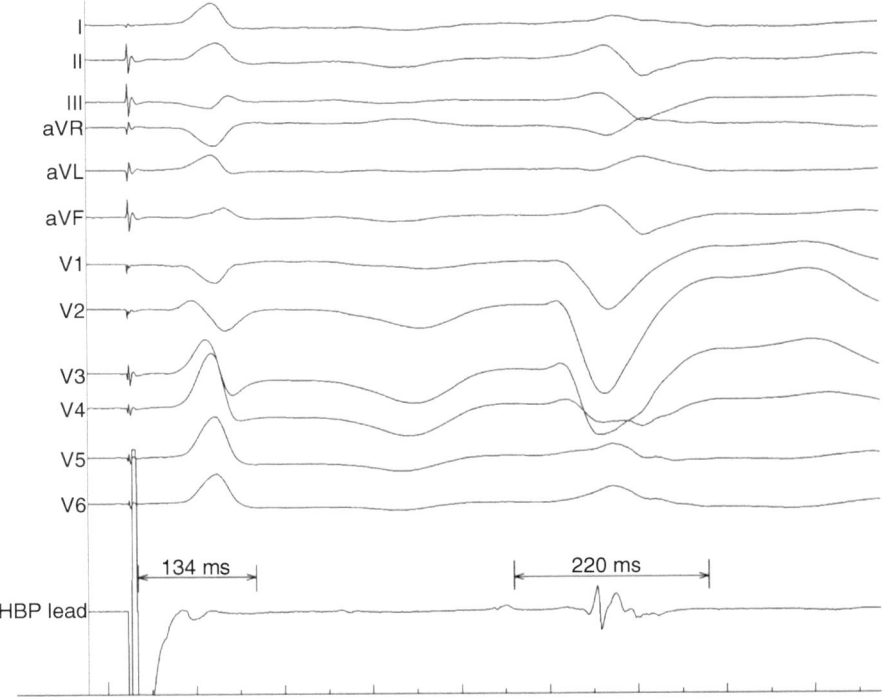

Fig. 7.5 His bundle pacing with selective capture (first beat) as evident by isoelectric baseline between Stim and QRS onset. Compared to native conduction with LBBB (second beat), His capture results in narrowing of QRS and morphology change by activating the left bundle distal to the site of disease

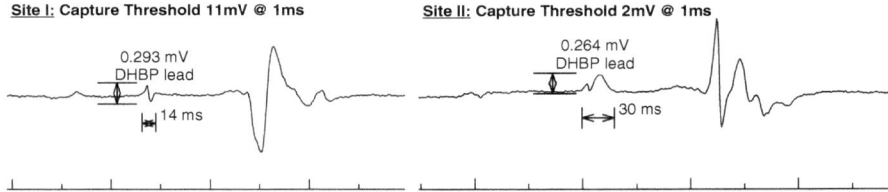

Fig. 7.6 Site 1 (proximal) – His potential, but high capture threshold (11 mV @ 1 ms). Site 2 (distal) – His potential with injury current, capture threshold at 2 mV @ 1 ms

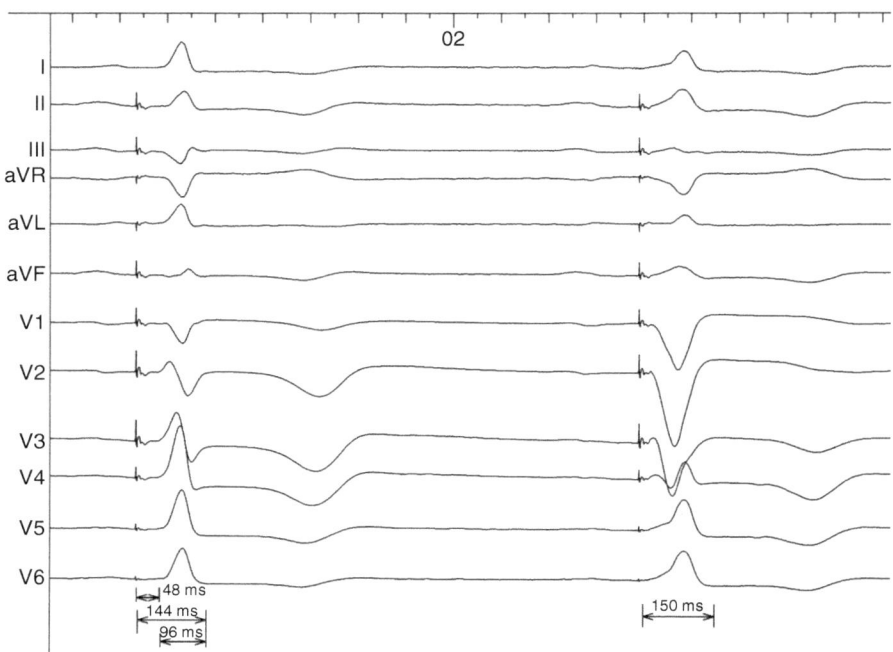

Fig. 7.7 Output-dependent His bundle capture. First beat (2 V @ 1 ms): Selective HBP with narrow QRS and isoelectric baseline between Stim and onset of QRS. Second beat (1.9 V @ 1 ms): Nonselective HBP with pseudo-delta wave due to capture of local ventricular myocardium as well as His capture

A His potential can be recorded at multiple sites along the membranous septum – suitability for pacing of a given site is determined by His to atrial amplitude and capture threshold (Fig. 7.6).

Figure 7.7 shows transition from selective to nonselective His bundle capture as the output is decreased from 2 V to 1.9 V at 1 ms. While nonselective capture has the benefit of ventricular capture as a safety factor should conduction disease progress distally or should AV node ablation without the use of a ventricular backup lead be planned, in some instances it can result in QRS widening and interventricular dyssynchrony.

Case II

An 81-year-old male with ischemic cardiomyopathy (LVEF 30% and LBBB) under-went CRT-D with a quadripolar LV lead. Unfortunately, he had intermittent dia-phragmatic stimulation prompting device reprogramming which required higher battery use. The patient was referred for LV lead revision, but repositioning proved to be difficult and the decision was made to place a His bundle pacing lead instead. The His bundle was mapped (Fig. 7.8) and paced proximally, resulting in nonselec-tive His capture only (Fig. 7.9). A slightly more anterior location resulted in left bundle conduction with marked QRS narrowing (Fig. 7.10). The patient's func-tional capacity improved from class III to class I at 3 months of follow-up.

Fig. 7.8 Intrinsic conduction – QRS of 252 ms with LBBB

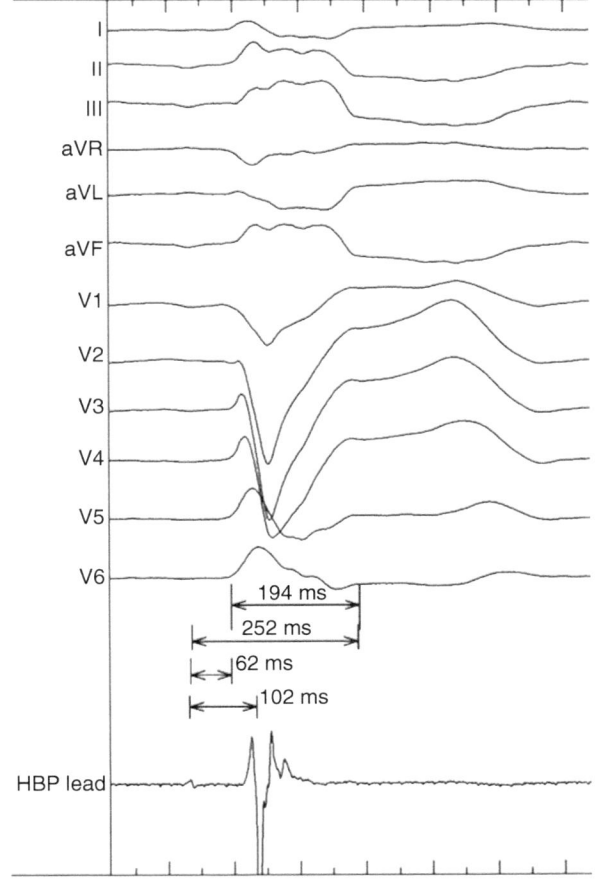

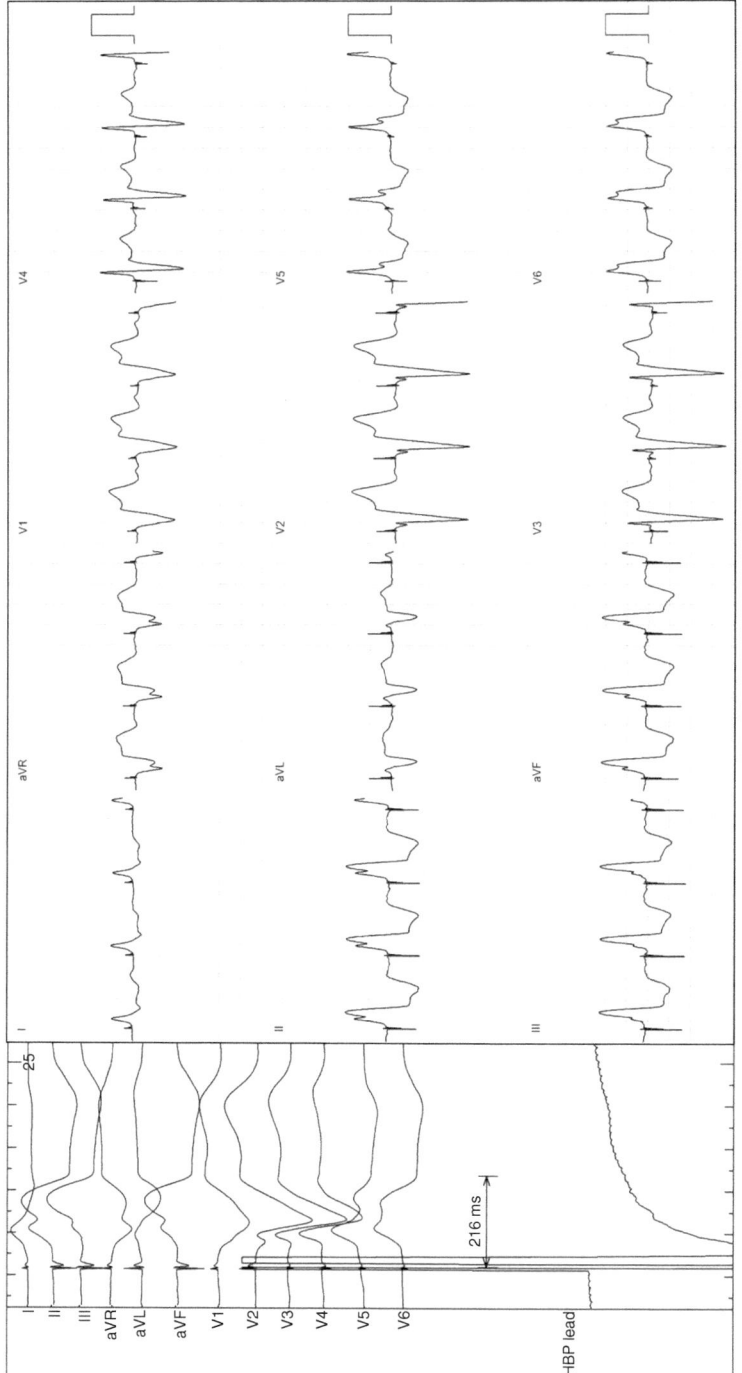

Fig. 7.9 Nonselective His bundle capture. QRS narrows as compared to baseline; however at this site, right ventricular excitation due to local ventricular capture from the His bundle lead is significant and may result in interventricular dyssynchrony

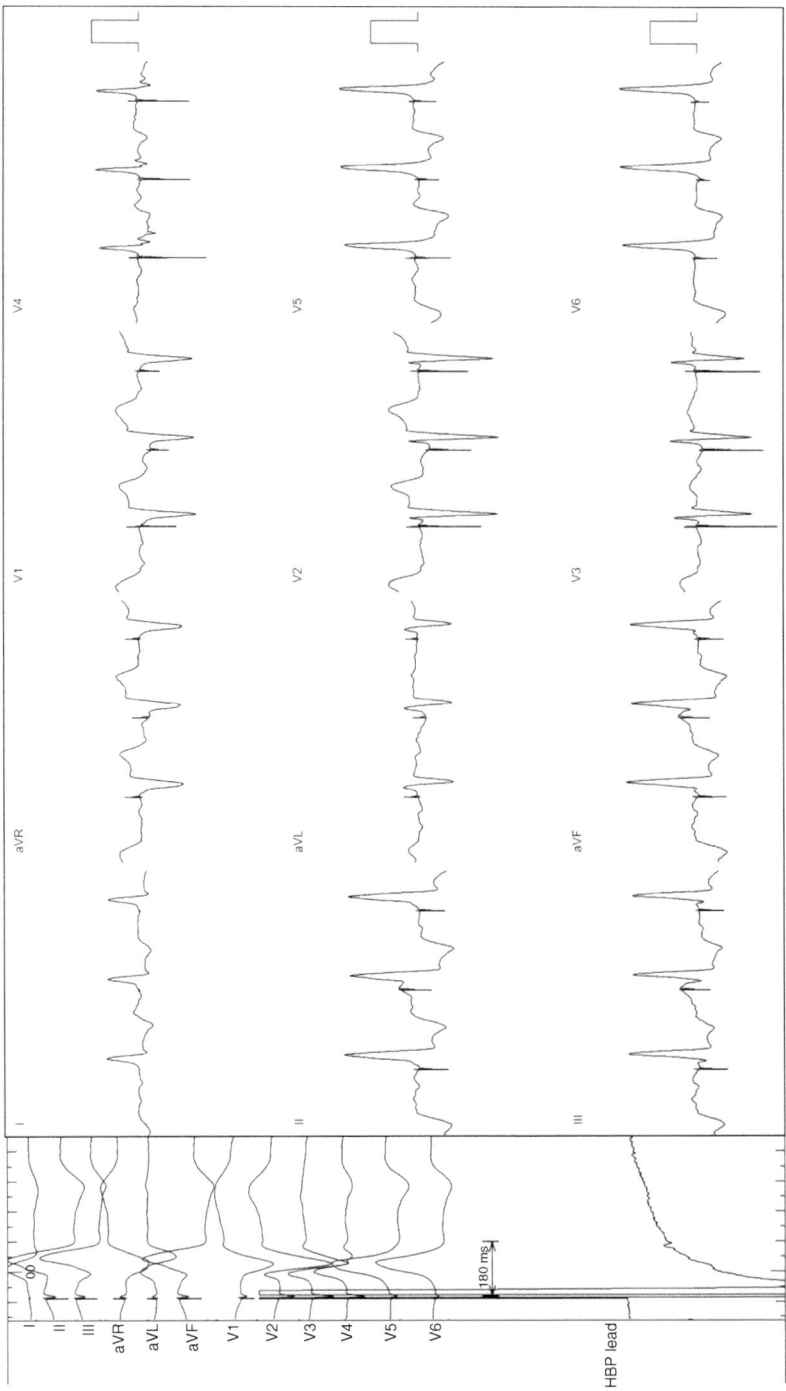

Fig. 7.10 Selective His bundle capture re-engages left bundle conduction and results in significant QRS narrowing

Future Directions

Ventricular resynchronization by engaging intact His-Purkinje fibers is conceptually superior to biventricular pacing, and outcomes data from multicenter experiences [38] are promising. However, randomized controlled trials are needed to compare efficacy of His bundle pacing vs. biventricular pacing, and until the publication of such data are available, His-CRT remains an option for patients who have for one reason or another failed the BiV-CRT option.

Procedural outcomes reported by Sharma et al. [30] illustrate a common trend with His bundle pacing: higher pacing thresholds with HBP (1.35 ± 0.9 V at the time of implantation and 1.50 ± 0.8 V at 2-year follow-up, 0.5 ms pulse width) as compared to RV pacing (0.62 ± 0.5 V at implantation and 0.80 ± 0.4 V at 2 years, 0.5 ms pulse width). In general, studies show stable long-term electrical performance of the His bundle lead; however in some cases, early device replacement has been required owing to high pacing output [34]. It is therefore important that further technical refinements in electrode design are pursued in order to achieve low stimulation thresholds. Optimizing tip electrode geometry is an important step toward that goal: a small electrode radius facilitates high impedance at the electrode-tissue interface (i.e., high current density), while porous or fractal coating increases the electrode's surface area, thereby minimizing polarization [39, 40]. Beyond refining lead design, enhancing sheath delivery systems and battery longevity are important components to improve care for patients requiring CRT.

References

1. Tracy CM, Epstein AE, Darbar D, et al. 2012 ACCF/AHA/HRS focused update of the 2008 guidelines for device-based therapy of cardiac rhythm abnormalities. J Thorac Cardiovasc Surg. 2012;144(6):e127–45.
2. Wiggers CJ. The muscular reaction of the mammalian ventricles to artificial surface stimuli. Am J Physiol – Leg Content. 1925;73(2):346–78.
3. Grines CL, Bashore TM, Boudoulas H, Olson S, Shafer P, Wooley CF. Functional abnormalities in isolated left bundle branch block. The effect of interventricular asynchrony. Circulation. 1989;79(4):845–53.
4. de Teresa E, Chamorro JL, Pulpón LA, et al. An even more physiological pacing: changing the sequence of ventricular activation, Cardiac Pacing. Heidelberg: Steinkopff; 1983. p. 395–400.
5. Bakker PF, Meijburg HW, de Vries JW, et al. Biventricular pacing in end-stage heart failure improves functional capacity and left ventricular function. J Interv Card Electrophysiol. 2000;4(2):395–404.
6. Daubert JC, Ritter P, Breton H, et al. Permanent left ventricular pacing with transvenous leads inserted into the coronary veins. Pacing Clin Electrophysiol. 1998;21(1):239–45.
7. Cazeau S, Leclercq C, Lavergne T, et al. Effects of multisite biventricular pacing in patients with heart failure and intraventricular conduction delay. N Engl J Med. 2001;344(12):873–80.
8. Abraham WT, Fisher WG, Smith AL, et al. Cardiac resynchronization in chronic heart failure. N Engl J Med. 2002;346(24):1845–53.
9. Bristow MR, Saxon LA, Boehmer J, et al. Cardiac-resynchronization therapy with or without an implantable defibrillator in advanced chronic heart failure. N Engl J Med. 2004;350(21):2140–50.

10. Cleland JGF, Daubert J-C, Erdmann E, et al. The effect of cardiac resynchronization on morbidity and mortality in heart failure. N Engl J Med. 2005;352(15):1539–49.
11. Moss AJ, Hall WJ, Cannom DS, et al. Cardiac-resynchronization therapy for the prevention of heart-failure events. N Engl J Med. 2009;361(14):1329–38.
12. Zareba W, Klein H, Cygankiewicz I, et al. Effectiveness of cardiac resynchronization therapy by QRS morphology in the Multicenter Automatic Defibrillator Implantation Trial–Cardiac Resynchronization Therapy (MADIT-CRT). Circulation. 2011;123(10):1061–72.
13. Gold MR, Thébault C, Linde C, et al. Effect of QRS duration and morphology on cardiac resynchronization therapy outcomes in mild heart failure. Circulation. 2012;126(7):822–9.
14. Stavrakis S, Lazzara R, Thadani U. The benefit of cardiac resynchronization therapy and QRS duration: a meta-analysis. J Cardiovasc Electrophysiol. 2012;23(2):163–8.
15. Biffi M, Moschini C, Bertini M, et al. Phrenic stimulation. Circ Arrhythmia Electrophysiol. 2009;2(4):402–10.
16. Durrer D, Vav Dam RT, Freud GE, Janse MJ, Meijler FL, Arzbaecher RC. Total excitation of the isolated human heart. Circulation. 1970;41(6):899–912.
17. Tomioka H, Liakopoulos OJ, Buckberg GD, Hristov N, Tan Z, Trummer G. The effect of ventricular sequential contraction on helical heart during pacing: high septal pacing versus biventricular pacing. Eur J Cardio-Thoracic Surg. 2006;29(Supplement_1):S198–206.
18. Tawara S. Das Reizleitungssystem des Säugetierherzens: eine anatomisch-histologische Studie über das Atrioventrikularbünel und die Purkinjeschen Fäden. Jena: Verlag von Gustav Fischer; 1906.
19. Suma K. Sunao Tawara: a father of modern cardiology. Pacing Clin Electrophysiol. 2001;24(1):88–96.
20. Kistin AD. Observations on the anatomy of the atrioventricular bundle (bundle of His) and the question of other muscular atrioventricular connections in normal human hearts. Am Heart J. 1949;37(6):849–67.
21. James TN. Structure and function of the sinus node, AV node and his bundle of the human heart: Part I—structure. Prog Cardiovasc Dis. 2002;45(3):235–67.
22. Kawashima T, Sasaki H. A macroscopic anatomical investigation of atrioventricular bundle locational variation relative to the membranous part of the ventricular septum in elderly human hearts. Surg Radiol Anat. 2005;27(3):206–13.
23. James TN, Sherf L. Fine structure of the his bundle. Circulation. 1971;44(1):9–28.
24. Narula OS. Longitudinal dissociation in the his bundle. Bundle branch block due to asynchronous conduction within the his bundle in man. Circulation. 1977;56(6):996–1006.
25. Scherlag BJ, Kosowsky BD, Damato AN. A technique for ventricular pacing from the His bundle of the intact heart. J Appl Physiol. 1967;22(3):584–7.
26. Narula OS, Scherlag BJ, Samet P. Pervenous pacing of the specialized conducting system in man. Circulation. 1970;41(1):77–87.
27. Deshmukh P, Casavant DA, Romanyshyn M, Anderson K. Permanent, direct His-Bundle pacing. Circulation. 2000;101(8):869–77.
28. Deshmukh PM, Romanyshyn M. Direct His-Bundle pacing: present and future. Pacing Clin Electrophysiol. 2004;27(6p2):862–70.
29. Zanon F, Baracca E, Aggio S, et al. A feasible approach for direct his-bundle pacing using a new steerable catheter to facilitate precise lead placement. J Cardiovasc Electrophysiol. 2006;17(1):29–33.
30. Sharma PS, Dandamudi G, Naperkowski A, et al. Permanent His-bundle pacing is feasible, safe, and superior to right ventricular pacing in routine clinical practice. Heart Rhythm. 2015;12(2):305–12.
31. Correa de Sa DD, Hardin NJ, Crespo EM, et al. Autopsy analysis of the implantation site of a permanent selective direct his bundle pacing lead. Circ Arrhythmia Electrophysiol. 2012;5(1):244–6.
32. Lustgarten D. Step-wise approach to permanent His Bundle pacing. J Innov Card Rhythm Manag. 2016;7(4):2313–21.

33. Catanzariti D, Maines M, Cemin C, Broso G, Marotta T, Vergara G. Permanent direct his bundle pacing does not induce ventricular dyssynchrony unlike conventional right ventricular apical pacing: an intrapatient acute comparison study. J Interv Card Electrophysiol. 2006;16(2):81–92.
34. Catanzariti D, Maines M, Manica A, Angheben C, Varbaro A, Vergara G. Permanent His-bundle pacing maintains long-term ventricular synchrony and left ventricular performance, unlike conventional right ventricular apical pacing. Europace. 2013;15(4):546–53.
35. Lustgarten DL, Calame S, Crespo EM, Calame J, Lobel R, Spector PS. Electrical resynchronization induced by direct His-bundle pacing. Heart Rhythm. 2010;7(1):15–21.
36. Lustgarten DL, Crespo EM, Arkhipova-Jenkins I, et al. His-bundle pacing versus biventricular pacing in cardiac resynchronization therapy patients: a crossover design comparison. Heart Rhythm. 2015;12(7):1548–57.
37. Sharma PS, Naperkowski A, Bauch TD, et al. Permanent His Bundle pacing for cardiac resynchronization therapy in patients with heart failure and right bundle branch block. Circ Arrhythmia Electrophysiol. 2018;11(9):e006613.
38. Sharma PS, Dandamudi G, Herweg B, et al. Permanent His-bundle pacing as an alternative to biventricular pacing for cardiac resynchronization therapy: a multicenter experience. Heart Rhythm. 2018;15(3):413–20.
39. Mond HG, Grenz D. Implantable Transvenous Pacing Leads: the shape of things to come. Pacing Clin Electrophysiol. 2004;27:887–93.
40. Ellenbogen KA, Wilkoff BL, Kay GN, Lau C-P, Auricchio A. Clinical cardiac pacing, defibrillation, and resynchronization therapy. 5th ed. Philadelphia: Elsevier; 2017.

Chapter 8
Replacement of Implantable Cardioverter-Defibrillators When Ventricular Function Has Recovered

Selcuk Adabag, Vidhu Anand, and Alejandra Gutierrez

Case Presentation

A 68-year-old man with a single-chamber implantable cardioverter-defibrillator (ICD) presented because his ICD was nearing the end of battery life. The ICD was implanted 6 years ago for primary prevention of sudden cardiac death (SCD). He has not had any appropriate ICD shocks. His left ventricular ejection fraction (EF), which was 30% at the time of ICD implantation, has improved to 45% since then. Is the ICD generator replacement justified?

ICD Generator Replacement Statistics

Approximately 30,000 ICD generator replacement procedures are performed in the United States annually for end of battery life, constituting 28% of all ICD procedures [1–3]. The most common reason for ICD generator replacement is the device

---

Drs. Anand and Gutierrez have contributed equally to the manuscript.

S. Adabag (✉)
Cardiology Division, Minneapolis Veterans Affairs Health Care System,
Minneapolis, MN, USA

Department of Cardiovascular Medicine, University of Minnesota, Minneapolis, MN, USA
e-mail: adaba001@umn.edu

V. Anand
Department of Cardiovascular Medicine, Mayo Clinic, Rochester, MN, USA

A. Gutierrez
Department of Cardiovascular Medicine, University of Minnesota, Minneapolis, MN, USA

reaching elective replacement indicator (ERI), an alert displayed by the ICD indicating that the battery may reach end of life in the next 3–6 months. It is recommended to replace the ICD generator within 3 months of reaching ERI. Other, less common reasons for replacing ICD generator are infection, upgrade to cardiac resynchronization therapy (CRT), lead or generator malfunction, and advisory recalls for increased risk of failure of ICD components [2–4].

Approximately, 65–70% of primary prevention ICD recipients remain free of appropriate ICD therapy during the lifetime of their initial ICD generator [2, 5, 6]. While it is common practice to routinely replace ICDs that reach ERI, a number of factors may limit the potential benefit of ICD after generator replacement. Patients presenting for ICD generator replacement tend to be older and have more comorbidities than those having initial ICD implant, increasing their competing risk of death from non-cardiovascular causes [1, 5, 7]. In a propensity-matched analysis of the National Cardiovascular Data Registry, survival after ICD replacement was worse compared to initial implant, regardless of device type [2].

Furthermore, ICD generator replacement procedure may be associated with significant complications such as infection, hematoma, or lead damage, which may result in increased morbidity and mortality [2, 8–10]. Indeed, patients presenting for an ICD generator replacement due to ERI have a periprocedural major complication rate of 4–6% [1, 5, 8, 9, 11]. Those who have a concomitant lead replacement have a 6-month complication rate of up to 15% [9]. The highest risk is associated with the need to replace a left ventricular lead with complication rates ranging from 9% to 50% [9].

The risk of mortality after ICD generator replacement is close to 10% at 1 year and up to 50% at 5 years [5, 7, 12–14]. Factors associated with higher mortality include increased age, atrial fibrillation, heart failure, worsened ejection fraction, chronic lung disease, diabetes, renal dysfunction, and history of stroke [1, 15]. Excessive long-term mortality in these cases is a testament to the higher-risk status of these patients rather than the risks of the ICD generator replacement procedure.

Implantable cardioverter-defibrillator generator replacement procedures also have a significant economic burden to the US healthcare system [16, 17]. The approximate cost of a single-chamber ICD replacement was around $18,000 in 2005 but increased to nearly $23,000 by 2013 [7, 18]. Thus, roughly $700 million is spent for ICD generator replacement in the USA each year.

While there is a close audit of indications at initial ICD implantation, routine reassessment of ICD indications is not mandated when these patients present for ICD generator replacement [6]. Identifying the patients who are least likely to benefit from continued ICD therapy may significantly reduce medical expenses by avoiding unnecessary ICD generator replacement.

Frequency of EF Improvement in Patients with ICD

Left ventricular EF is the cornerstone of the criteria used in the decision process to recommend or decline ICD implantation for primary prevention of SCD [19].

Professional society practice guideline statements recommend ICD implantation in patients with EF ≤35% and mild to moderate heart failure symptoms while taking optimal medical therapy [20–22]. The EF cut-off is based on randomized controlled trials, in which patients assigned to ICD and medical therapy were more likely to survive compared to those assigned to medical therapy alone. However, patients presenting for ICD generator replacement have a left ventricular EF that is, on average, 4–5% higher than it had been at the time of the initial ICD implantation [1, 5]. As such, 25–40% of the patients who receive an ICD for primary prevention of SCD experience an improvement in their EF to the extent that they are no longer eligible for ICD therapy when they present for generator replacement. The proportion of patients with EF improvement has been consistent in cohorts that include ICD alone and those that also include CRT [14, 23].

Patients who experience an improvement in EF are younger, more likely to be women, more likely to be taking heart failure medications, and, most notably, more likely to have nonischemic cardiomyopathy [14, 23]. They also have less comorbidity, smaller left ventricular volume, and lower body mass index [24, 25]. Cardiomyopathy due to reversible causes such as tachycardia, myocarditis, pregnancy, hyperthyroidism, stress, pacing, or alcohol is more likely to improve after the offending etiology is treated or eliminated. Thus, 50% of the individuals with nonischemic cardiomyopathy assigned to ICD in the DEFINITE (Defibrillators in Nonischemic Cardiomyopathy Treatment Evaluation) trial experienced a significant (>5% absolute) improvement in EF [13]. In comparison, 20–25% of the patients with ischemic cardiomyopathy experience improvement in EF [26, 27]. Medical therapies and revascularization have been associated with improvement in EF in ischemic cardiomyopathy [28–33]. In addition to the factors associated with a higher likelihood of EF improvement, patients with a baseline EF in the range of 30–35% at the time of ICD implantation are more likely to be ineligible for ICD at the time of battery depletion [7, 26]. These data show that EF improvement is common after ICD implantation and 25–40% of the patients who qualified for ICD on the basis of a low EF will no longer be eligible for ICD implantation by the time they present for generator replacement.

Appropriate ICD Therapy After EF Improvement

With improvement in EF, the incidence of appropriate ICD therapy is reduced but not completely eliminated (Table 8.1) [5, 7, 12–14, 26, 34–41]. In recent cohort studies, improvement in EF was associated with a 70% reduction in the risk of appropriate ICD therapy, which ranged from 2.8% to 5% per year (Fig. 8.1) [5, 7, 14]. Conversely, two earlier studies had found a similar incidence of appropriate ICD shock among patients with improved or unchanged EF [13, 26]. The reason for the dissimilar results in these studies may have been aggressive ICD programming parameters, which have evolved over the years to reduce shocks delivered for arrhythmias that are likely to terminate spontaneously [42].

Table 8.1 Description of the studies assessing the outcomes of patients with and without improvement in left ventricular ejection fraction after defibrillator implantation

Author year	N	Device type	Primary or secondary prevention	Cardiomyopathy	EF improvement criteria	Improved EF	Appropriate ICD therapy improved vs. unchanged EF	Mortality improved vs. unchanged EF
Schaer (2010) [39]	221	ICD or CRT	Primary or secondary	Nonischemic	EF >35%	ICD 44.9% CRT 22.5%	28.3% vs. 43.9%	No data
Barsheshet (2011) [40]	749	CRT	Primary	Ischemic or nonischemic	>25% reduction in LVESV from baseline	70.6%	12% vs. 28%	15% vs. 35%
Naksuk (2013) [26]	91	ICD	Primary	Ischemic or nonischemic	EF >35% and >10% improvement from baseline	27%	28% vs. 26%	No data
Manfredi (2013) [12]	357	CRT	Primary or secondary	Ischemic or nonischemic	EF >45%	16.2%	6.9% vs. 20%	No data
Schliamser (2013) [13]	187	ICD	Primary	Nonischemic	>5% improvement in EF from baseline	51.3%	17.3% vs. 13.2%	3.1% vs. 15%
Sebag (2014) [34]	107	CRT	Primary or secondary	Ischemic or nonischemic	EF ≥40%	45%	5% vs. 28%	No data
Kini (2014) [7]	231	ICD or CRT	Primary	Ischemic or nonischemic	EF >40%	26%	8% vs. 38%	No data
Zhang (2015) [14]	538	ICD or CRT	Primary	Ischemic or nonischemic	>5% improvement in EF from baseline or EF >35%	40% (EF improved >5% from baseline) 25% (EF >35%)	3.0% vs. 7.8% (by >5% criterion) or 3.1% vs. 6.8% (by >35% criterion)	7.9% vs. 24% (by >5% criterion)
Kawata (2016) [35]	168	ICD	Primary	Ischemic or nonischemic	EF >35%	47%	11.6 vs. 56.8	No data
Madhavan (2016) [5]	253	ICD	Primary	Ischemic or nonischemic	EF >35%	28%	5%/year vs. 12%/year	5% vs. 7%
House (2016) [36]	125	ICD or CRT	Primary	Ischemic or nonischemic	EF >35%	44%	9% vs. 14%	No data
Madeira (2017) [37]	121	ICD or CRT	Primary or secondary	Ischemic or nonischemic	EF >35%	36%	2.6% vs. 32.9%	10.3% vs. 26.8%
Weng (2017) [38]	173	CRT or ICD	Primary	Ischemic or nonischemic	EF >35%	19%	17.2% vs. 33.3%	17.2% vs. 28.5%
Adabag (2017) [41]	624	ICD	Primary	Ischemic or nonischemic	EF >35%	29.8%	No data	6% vs. 20%

CRT cardiac resynchronization therapy, EF ejection fraction, ICD implantable cardioverter-defibrillator

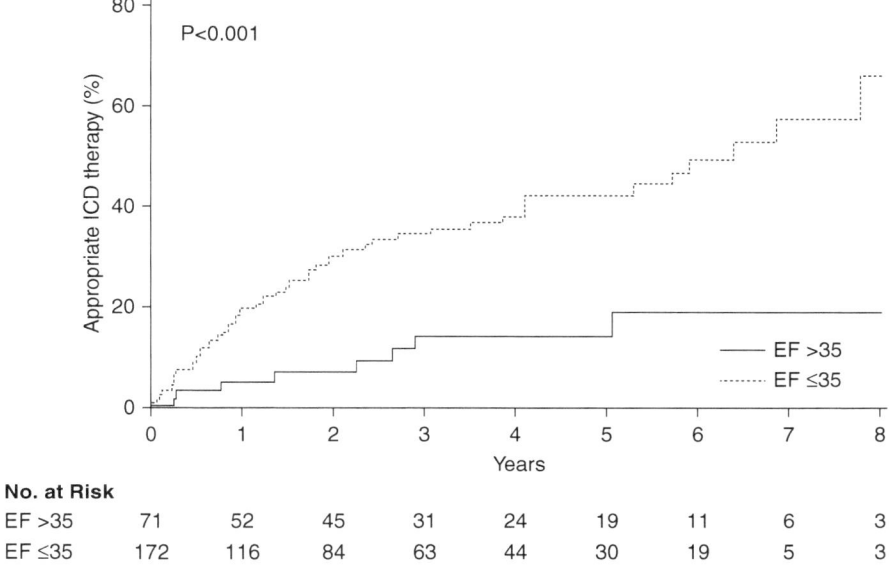

Fig. 8.1 Cumulative incidence of appropriate ICD therapy after generator replacement among patients with or without EF improvement. (Adopted with permission from Madhavan et al. [5])

Absence of appropriate ICD therapy before generator replacement is not a sufficient reassurance for not having future ICD therapies. Approximately, 20% of patients who had an improvement in EF and no prior appropriate ICD therapies experience their first appropriate ICD therapy after generator replacement [26]. In a cohort study of such patients, the incidence of ICD therapy was 5% per year [5].

Patients with normalized EF constitute a special subgroup of EF improvement. These patients either have a reversible cardiomyopathy or can be classified as super responders to CRT. Super responders to CRT have a similar mortality risk to the general population [12, 40, 43]. Although the risk of appropriate ICD shocks decreases markedly in patients with normalized EF, a small risk remains. In a prospective cohort study by Zhang et al., only 1 of the 35 patients with normalized EF had an appropriate ICD shock during follow-up (1.7 shock/100 person-years) [14]. On the other hand, none of the 18 patients with EF >55% after CRT in a series by Manfredi et al. had appropriate ICD therapy [12].

Patients with CRT are more likely to experience improvement and normalization of LVEF compared to patients with ICD [14]. However, the association between changes in left ventricular EF and ICD therapy appears to be similar in ICD and CRT, suggesting that the improvement in EF itself, but not the means that caused the improvement, is responsible from the favorable results [14].

Collectively, these data show that 20–30% of patients with EF improvement are at risk of receiving appropriate ICD shock/therapy, but the risk appears to be lower as the EF approaches normal range. The persisting risk of arrhythmias, observed in some patients despite improvement in EF, may be partly explained by the presence of a fixed substrate for ventricular arrhythmias (e.g., fibrosis, myocardial scar, heterogeneous repolarization) that does not resolve even when EF improves [14, 44–49]. However, the other factors associated with a persisting risk of SCD in patients with improved EF are presently unknown.

Do ICDs Reduce Mortality After Improvement of EF?

Left ventricular EF is a major determinant of arrhythmic and non-arrhythmic mortality [50]. Thus, it should come as no surprise that improvement in EF among patients with ICD is associated with improved survival in comparison with unchanged EF in the great majority of the cohort studies to date (Table 8.1). However, because of a lack of a control group without ICD, these cohort studies cannot determine whether ICD improves the likelihood of survival in patients with an improvement in EF. In the absence of prospective randomized controlled trials, we assessed the efficacy of ICD in prolonging survival among patients with improved EF in a secondary analysis of the Sudden Cardiac Death in Heart Failure Trial (SCD-HeFT) [41]. The SCD-HeFT was a randomized controlled trial of ICD, amiodarone, or placebo among 2511 patients with heart failure symptoms and EF ≤35% due to ischemic or nonischemic cardiomyopathy [51]. After a median 45.5 months of follow-up, the patients assigned to ICD had a lower likelihood of mortality than those assigned to placebo or amiodarone (22%, 29%, and 28%, respectively), resulting in a 23% reduction in the relative risk and a 7.2% reduction in the absolute risk of mortality in comparison with the placebo group. While not mandated by the study protocol, nearly 75% of the patients in SCD-HeFT had a repeated assessment of EF 1 year after enrollment. Of these, 30% assigned to ICD or placebo showed a significant improvement in EF where the mean EF increased from 27% to 45%. During a median follow-up of 30 months after the repeated EF measurement, all-cause mortality rate was lower in the ICD vs. placebo groups both in patients whose EF improved to levels >35% (2.6% vs. 4.5% per 100-person-year follow-up, respectively) and in those whose EF remained ≤35% (7.7% vs. 10.7% per 100-person-year follow-up, respectively) (Fig. 8.2). Compared with placebo, the adjusted hazard ratio for the effect of ICD on mortality was 0.64 (95% CI, 0.48–0.85) in patients with repeated EF ≤35% and 0.62 (95% CI, 0.29–1.30) in those with a repeated EF >35% (Table 8.2). There was no interaction between treatment assignment and repeated EF for predicting mortality, suggesting that the efficacy of ICD was similar in patients with improved or unchanged EF. Cumulatively, these results suggest that mortality is lower among patients with improved EF, but ICD remains effective in reducing all-cause mortality among these patients.

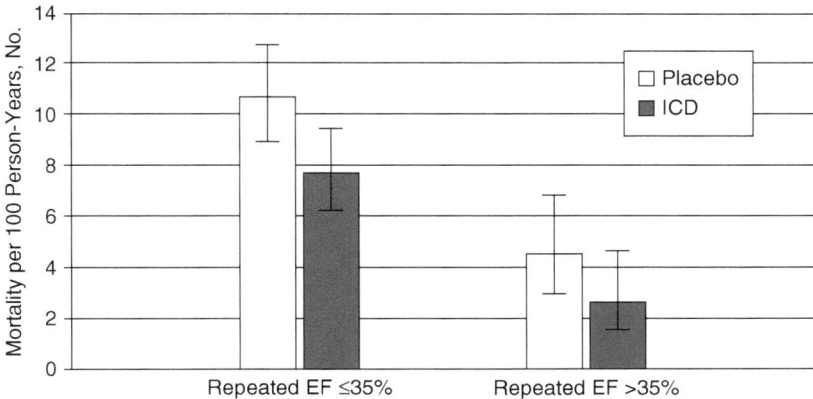

Fig. 8.2 Incidence rate of all-cause mortality of patients assigned to ICD vs. placebo. Adjusted hazard ratios of all-cause mortality in the ICD vs the placebo groups were 0.64 (95% CI, 0.48–0.85) in patients with a repeated ejection fraction (EF) ≤35% and 0.62 (95% CI, 0.29–1.30) in those with an EF >35%. (Adopted with permission from Adabag et al. [41])

Table 8.2 Incidence rates of all-cause mortality and SCD in the ICD and control groups in each EF category

EF Group	No. Patients	Deaths	100 Follow-up Person-years	Incidence Rate Mortality per 100 Person-year Follow-up (95% CI)
All-Cause Mortality				
EF ≤35%				
ICD	438	89	11.5	7.7 (6.3-9.5)
Placebo	464	125	11.7	10.7 (8.9-12.7)
EF > 35%				
ICD	186	12	4.6	2.6 (1.5-4.6)
Placebo	185	22	4.9	4.5 (3.0-6.8)
SCD				
EF ≤ 35%				
ICD	438	14	11.5	1.2 (0.7-2.0)
Placebo	464	46	11.7	3.9 (2.9-5.2)
EF > 35%				
ICD	186	3	4.6	0.6 (0.2-2.0)
Placebo	185	4	4.9	0.8 (0.3-2.2)

Abbreviations: EF, ejection fraction; ICD, implantable cardioverter defibrillator; SCD, sudden cardiac death.

Proposed Algorithm

Patients who present for ICD generator replacement should be reevaluated for the appropriateness of continued ICD therapy (Fig. 8.3). The evaluation should first exclude any potential contraindications, such as advanced malignancy, that may have developed since the initial implant. A repeat echocardiogram to assess left ventricular function is prudent, if one has not been performed since the initial ICD implantation. A frank discussion to learn the patient's values and wishes about continued ICD therapy is of utmost importance to help guide the decision and to clarify potential misconceptions.

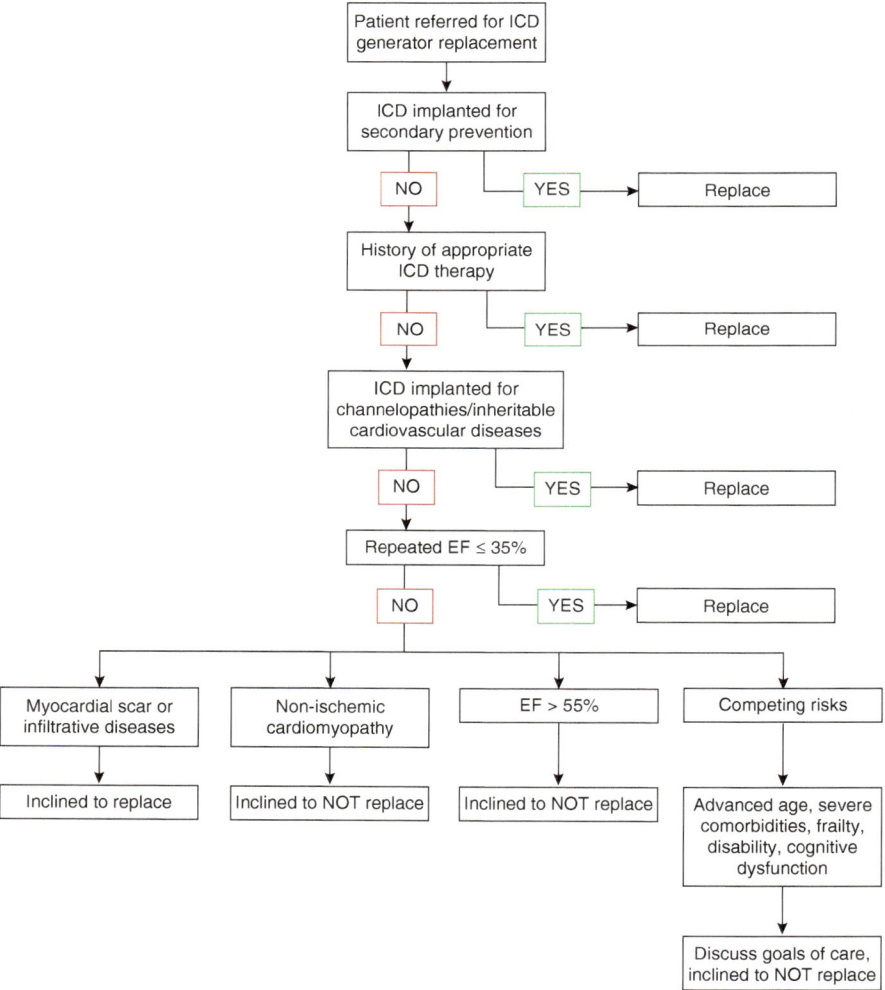

Fig. 8.3 Recommended algorithm for patients who present for ICD generator replacement

We recommend replacement of the generator if the original indication for ICD was secondary prevention of SCD. The risk of appropriate ICD therapy is higher (10%/year versus 5%/year) if the ICD was implanted for secondary prevention of SCD [52].

We also recommend generator replacement if there was an appropriate ICD therapy (shock or antitachycardia pacing) during the lifetime of the initial device. In addition to the host factors such as the rate and frequency of the ventricular tachycardia/ventricular fibrillation, the likelihood of appropriate ICD shocks also depends on the programmed tachycardia therapy parameters with a rise in the likelihood with more aggressive programming schemes. Indeed, it has been well documented that some ICD shocks for ventricular tachycardia/ventricular fibrillation are delivered prematurely for arrhythmias that would have terminated anyway. While we support utilization of newer ICD programming schemes to prevent inappropriate and appropriate—but unnecessary—shocks, we also recommend replacing the ICD generator in patients with prior appropriate ICD shock because of the increased risk of future shocks in these patients.

We also recommend generator replacement in patients with channelopathies/inheritable arrhythmogenic syndromes due to the continuation of risk. Similarly, patients whose EF remains ≤35% continue to be at SCD risk and should undergo generator replacement.

On the other hand, some patients who are no longer eligible for ICD due to improvement in EF deserve a fair discussion of whether the SCD risk warrants continuation of ICD therapy. Patients with nonischemic cardiomyopathy have a lower risk of SCD and may not benefit from ongoing ICD therapy if EF has improved [53, 54]. Patients with normalized EF (>55%) may also not benefit from continued ICD therapy [12, 14, 40, 43]. On the other hand, patients with a prior myocardial scar may continue to benefit from ICD even if their EF is better [49].

Older patients who have developed competing risks of death due to new comorbidities (e.g., renal failure) or those with frailty, disability, or cognitive dysfunction should have an opportunity to reevaluate continued ICD therapy with an extensive discussion of goals of care [55, 56]. In cases with difficulty in assessing risk additional markers such as inducibility of ventricular tachycardia, or magnetic resonance imaging to identify and quantify fibrosis may be useful [5, 57].

Management of Unreplaced ICDs

There is very limited data on whether or not to explant the ICD that has reached ERI and does not need replacement. Some device manufacturers recommend explanting the ICD to avoid any potential harm from erratic device behavior. The rationale for this recommendation comes from the concern that as the battery continues to deplete, the performance of the transistors (electrical switches) within the ICD may become unpredictable due to the lack of current supplied to these components, which control a number of functions including sensing, pacing, and shock delivery. However, other manufacturers note that at battery depletion, the ICD will revert to storage mode in which no functionality is present. Thus, although no data are available, it is very unlikely for an ICD at the end of life to be able to generate enough power to deliver a shock. Indeed, in our limited experience, patients prefer leaving the device in order to avoid the burden and stress of the explant procedure. In two anecdotal cases, we have left the device without any negative clinical consequences.

However, patients with CRT defibrillator constitute a special situation. Even if the decision is made *not* to replace a CRT defibrillator, the device, in most instances, should be replaced with a CRT pacemaker to continue synchronization of the left ventricle, particularly if the patient is a "responder" to CRT. Similarly, among patients with a pacing indication who do not wish continued ICD therapy, the ICD should be replaced with a pacemaker [58, 59].

References

1. Kramer DB, Kennedy KF, Spertus JA, Normand SL, Noseworthy PA, Buxton AE, Josephson ME, Zimetbaum PJ, Mitchell SL, Reynolds MR. Mortality risk following replacement implantable cardioverter-defibrillator implantation at end of battery life: results from the NCDR. Heart Rhythm. 2014;11(2):216–21. PMID: 24513917.
2. Kramer DB, Kennedy KF, Noseworthy PA, Buxton AE, Josephson ME, Normand SL, Spertus JA, Zimetbaum PJ, Reynolds MR, Mitchell SL. Characteristics and outcomes of patients receiving new and replacement implantable cardioverter-defibrillators: results from the NCDR. Circ Cardiovasc Qual Outcomes. 2013;6(4):488–97. PMID: 23759471.
3. Merchant FM, Quest T, Leon AR, El-Chami MF. Implantable cardioverter-defibrillators at end of battery life: opportunities for risk (re)-stratification in ICD recipients. J Am Coll Cardiol. 2016;67(4):435–44. PMID: 26821633.
4. Gakenheimer L, Romero J, Baman TS, Montgomery D, Smith CA, Oral H, Eagle KA, Crawford T. Cardiac implantable electronic device reutilization: battery life of explanted devices at a tertiary care center. Pacing Clin Electrophysiol. 2014;37(5):569–75. PMID: 24359248.
5. Madhavan M, Waks JW, Friedman PA, Kramer DB, Buxton AE, Noseworthy PA, Mehta RA, Hodge DO, Higgins AY, Webster TL, Witt CM, Cha YM, Gersh BJ. Outcomes after implantable cardioverter-defibrillator generator replacement for primary prevention of sudden cardiac death. Circ Arrhythm Electrophysiol. 2016;9(3):e003283. PMID: 26921377.
6. Kramer DB, Buxton AE, Zimetbaum PJ. Time for a change—a new approach to ICD replacement. N Engl J Med. 2012;366(4):291–3. PMID: 22276818.
7. Kini V, Soufi MK, Deo R, Epstein AE, Bala R, Riley M, Groeneveld PW, Shalaby A, Dixit S. Appropriateness of primary prevention implantable cardioverter-defibrillators at the time of generator replacement: are indications still met? J Am Coll Cardiol. 2014;63(22):2388–94. PMID: 24727249.
8. Krahn AD, Lee DS, Birnie D, Healey JS, Crystal E, Dorian P, Simpson CS, Khaykin Y, Cameron D, Janmohamed A, Yee R, Austin PC, Chen Z, Hardy J, Tu JV, Ontario ICD Database Investigators. Predictors of short-term complications after implantable cardioverter-defibrillator replacement: results from the Ontario ICD database. Circ Arrhythm Electrophysiol. 2011;4(2):136–42. PMID: 21325209.
9. Poole JE, Gleva MJ, Mela T, Chung MK, Uslan DZ, Borge R, Gottipaty V, Shinn T, Dan D, Feldman LA, Seide H, Winston SA, Gallagher JJ, Langberg JJ, Mitchell K, Holcomb R, REPLACE Registry Investigators. Complication rates associated with pacemaker or implantable cardioverter-defibrillator generator replacements and upgrade procedures: results from the REPLACE registry. Circulation. 2010;122(16):1553–61. PMID: 20921437.

10. Lovelock JD, Cruz C, Hoskins MH, Jones P, El-Chami MF, Lloyd MS, Leon A, DeLurgio DB, Langberg JJ. Generator replacement is associated with an increased rate of ICD lead alerts. Heart Rhythm. 2014;11(10):1785–9. PMID: 24953380.
11. Gould PA, Krahn AD, Canadian Heart Rhythm Society Working Group on Device Advisories. Complications associated with implantable cardioverter-defibrillator replacement in response to device advisories. JAMA. 2006;295(16):1907–11. PMID: 16639049.
12. Manfredi JA, Al-Khatib SM, Shaw LK, Thomas L, Fogel RI, Padanilam B, Rardon D, Vatthyam R, Gemma LW, Golden K, Prystowsky EN. Association between left ventricular ejection fraction post-cardiac resynchronization treatment and subsequent implantable cardioverter defibrillator therapy for sustained ventricular tachyarrhythmias. Circ Arrhythm Electrophysiol. 2013;6(2):257–64. PMID: 23443618.
13. Schliamser JE, Kadish AH, Subacius H, Shalaby A, Schaechter A, Levine J, Goldberger JJ, DEFINITE Investigators. Significance of follow-up left ventricular ejection fraction measurements in the Defibrillators in Non-Ischemic Cardiomyopathy Treatment Evaluation trail (DEFINITE). Heart Rhythm. 2013;10(6):838–46. PMID: 23422221.
14. Zhang Y, Guallar E, Blasco-Colmenares E, Butcher B, Norgard S, Nauffal V, Marine JE, Eldadah Z, Dickfeld T, Ellenbogen KA, Tomaselli GF, Cheng A. Changes in follow-up left ventricular ejection fraction associated with outcomes in primary prevention implantable cardioverter-defibrillator and cardiac resynchronization therapy device recipients. J Am Coll Cardiol. 2015;66(5):524–31. PMID: 26227190.
15. Voight J, Akkaya M, Somasundaram P, Karim R, Valliani S, Kwon Y, Adabag S. Risk of new-onset atrial fibrillation and stroke after radiofrequency ablation of isolated, typical atrial flutter. Heart Rhythm. 2014;11(11):1884–9. PMID: 24998999.
16. Hospital outpatient prospective payment – final rule with comment period and CY2013 payment rates. Centers for Medicare & Medicaid Services, Jan 18, 2011. http://www.cms.gov/Medicare/Medicare-Fee-for-Service-Payment/HospitalOutpatientPPS/Hospital-Outpatient-Regulations-and-Notices-Items/CMS-1589-FC.html.
17. Physician fee schedule. Centers for Medicare & Medicaid Services, July 12, 2018. https://www.cms.gov/Medicare/Medicare-Fee-for-Service-Payment/PhysicianFeeSched/index.html.
18. Sanders GD, Hlatky MA, Owens DK. Cost-effectiveness of implantable cardioverter-defibrillators. N Engl J Med. 2005;353(14):1471–80. PMID: 16207849.
19. Adabag S, Hodgson L, Garcia S, Anand V, Frascone R, Conterato M, Lick C, Wesley K, Mahoney B, Yannopoulos D. Outcomes of sudden cardiac arrest in a state-wide integrated resuscitation program: results from the Minnesota Resuscitation Consortium. Resuscitation. 2017;110:95–100. PMID: 27865744.
20. Al-Khatib SM, Stevenson WG, Ackerman MJ, Gillis AM, Bryant WJ, Hlatky MA, Callans DJ, Granger CB, Curtis AB, Hammill SC, Deal BJ, Joglar JA, Dickfeld T, Kay GN, Field ME, Matlock DD, Fonarow GC, Myerburg RJ, Page RL. 2017 AHA/ACC/HRS guideline for management of patients with ventricular arrhythmias and the prevention of sudden cardiac death: executive summary: a report of the American College of Cardiology/American Heart Association Task Force on Clinical Practice Guidelines and the Heart Rhythm Society. Heart rhythm J 2018;15(10): e73–e189.
21. Vakil K, Kazmirczak F, Sathnur N, Adabag S, Cantillon DJ, Kiehl EL, Koene R, Cogswell R, Anand I, Roukoz H. Implantable cardioverter-defibrillator use in patients with left ventricular assist device: a systematic review and meta-analysis. JACC Heart Fail. 2016;4(10):772–9. PMID: 27395347.
22. Vakil K, Duval S, Cogswell R, Eckman P, Levy WC, Anand I, Dardas T, Adabag S. Impact of implantable cardioverter-defibrillators on waitlist mortality among patients awaiting heart transplantation: an UNOS/OPTN analysis. JACC Clin Electrophysiol. 2017;3(1):33–40. PMID: 29759692.
23. Smer A, Saurav A, Azzouz MS, Salih M, Ayan M, Abuzaid A, Akinapelli A, Kanmanthareddy A, Rosenfeld LE, Merchant FM, Abuissa H. Meta-analysis of risk of ventricular arrhythmias after improvement in left ventricular ejection fraction during follow-up in patients with primary prevention implantable cardioverter defibrillators. Am J Cardiol. 2017;120(2):279–86. PMID: 28532779.

24. Pires LA, Ghio S, Chung ES, Tavazzi L, Abraham WT, Gerritse B. Relationship between acute improvement in left ventricular function to 6-month outcomes after cardiac resynchronization therapy in patients with chronic heart failure. Congest Heart Fail. 2011;17(2):65–70. PMID: 21449994.

25. Hsu JC, Solomon SD, Bourgoun M, McNitt S, Goldenberg I, Klein H, Moss AJ, Foster E, MADIT-CRT Executive Committee. Predictors of super-response to cardiac resynchronization therapy and associated improvement in clinical outcome: the MADIT-CRT (multicenter automatic defibrillator implantation trial with cardiac resynchronization therapy) study. J Am Coll Cardiol. 2012;59(25):2366–73. PMID: 22698490.

26. Naksuk N, Saab A, Li JM, Florea V, Akkaya M, Anand IS, Benditt DG, Adabag S. Incidence of appropriate shock in implantable cardioverter-defibrillator patients with improved ejection fraction. J Card Fail. 2013;19(6):426–30. PMID: 23743493.

27. Naksuk N, Adabag S. What to do about primary-prevention implantable cardiac defibrillators in patients with improved ejection fraction. Curr Heart Fail Rep. 2014;11(2):197–200. PMID: 24500435.

28. Cintron G, Johnson G, Francis G, Cobb F, Cohn JN. Prognostic significance of serial changes in left ventricular ejection fraction in patients with congestive heart failure. The V-HeFT VA Cooperative Studies Group. Circulation. 1993;87(6 Suppl):VI17–23. PMID: 8500235.

29. Konstam MA, Rousseau MF, Kronenberg MW, Udelson JE, Melin J, Stewart D, Dolan N, Edens TR, Ahn S, Kinan D, et al. Effects of the angiotensin converting enzyme inhibitor enalapril on the long-term progression of left ventricular dysfunction in patients with heart failure. SOLVD Investigators. Circulation. 1992;86(2):431–8. PMID: 1638712.

30. Packer M, Colucci WS, Sackner-Bernstein JD, Liang CS, Goldscher DA, Freeman I, Kukin ML, Kinhal V, Udelson JE, Klapholz M, Gottlieb SS, Pearle D, Cody RJ, Gregory JJ, Kantrowitz NE, LeJemtel TH, Young ST, Lukas MA, Shusterman NH. Double-blind, placebo-controlled study of the effects of carvedilol in patients with moderate to severe heart failure. The PRECISE Trial. Prospective Randomized Evaluation of Carvedilol on Symptoms and Exercise. Circulation. 1996;94(11):2793–9. PMID: 8941104.

31. Adabag S, Roukoz H, Anand IS, Moss AJ. Cardiac resynchronization therapy in patients with minimal heart failure: a systematic review and meta-analysis. J Am Coll Cardiol. 2011;58(9):935–41. PMID: 21851882.

32. St John Sutton MG, Plappert T, Abraham WT, Smith AL, DeLurgio DB, Leon AR, Loh E, Kocovic DZ, Fisher WG, Ellestad M, Messenger J, Kruger K, Hilpisch KE, Hill MR, Multicenter InSync Randomized Clinical Evaluation (MIRACLE) Study Group. Effect of cardiac resynchronization therapy on left ventricular size and function in chronic heart failure. Circulation. 2003;107(15):1985–90. PMID: 12668512.

33. Vakil K, Florea V, Koene R, Kealhofer JV, Anand I, Adabag S. Effect of coronary artery bypass grafting on left ventricular ejection fraction in men eligible for implantable cardioverter-defibrillator. Am J Cardiol. 2016;117(6):957–60. PMID: 26803382.

34. Sebag FA, Lellouche N, Chen Z, Tritar A, O'Neill MD, Gill J, Wright M, Leclercq C, Rinaldi CA. Positive response to cardiac resynchronization therapy reduces arrhythmic events after elective generator change in patients with primary prevention CRT-D. J Cardiovasc Electrophysiol. 2014;25(12):1368–75. PMID: 25066404.

35. Kawata H, Hirai T, Doukas D, Hirai R, Steinbrunner J, Wilson J, Noda T, Hsu J, Krummen D, Feld G, Wilber D, Santucci P, Birgersdotter-Green U. The occurrence of implantable cardioverter defibrillator therapies after generator replacement in patients who no longer meet primary prevention indications. J Cardiovasc Electrophysiol. 2016;27(6):724–9. PMID: 26915696.

36. House CM, Nguyen D, Thomas AJ, Nelson WB, Zhu DW. Normalization of left ventricular ejection fraction and incidence of appropriate antitachycardia therapy in patients with implantable cardioverter defibrillator for primary prevention of sudden death. J Card Fail. 2016;22(2):125–32. PMID: 26522819.

37. Madeira M, António N, Milner J, Ventura M, Cristóvão J, Costa M, Nascimento J, Elvas L, Gonçalves L, Mariano Pego G. Who still remains at risk of arrhythmic death at time of implantable cardioverter-defibrillator generator replacement? Pacing Clin Electrophysiol. 2017;40(10):1129–38. PMID: 28842918.

38. Weng W, Sapp J, Doucette S, MacIntyre C, Gray C, Gardner M, Abdelwahab A, Parkash R. Benefit of implantable cardioverter-defibrillator generator replacement in a primary prevention population-based cohort. JACC Clin Electrophysiol. 2017;3(10):1180–9. PMID: 29759503.

39. Schaer B, Theuns DA, Stitcherling C, Szili-Torok T, Osswald S, Jordaens L. Effect of implantable cardioverter-defibrillator on left ventricular ejection fraction in patients with idiopathic dilated cardiomyopathy. Am J Cardiol. 2010;106(11):1640–5. PMID: 21094367.

40. Barsheshet A, Wang PJ, Moss AJ, Solomon SD, Al-Ahmad A, McNitt S, Foster E, Huang DT, Klein HU, Zareba W, Eldar M, Goldenberg I. Reverse remodeling and the risk of ventricular tachyarrhythmias in the MADIT-CRT (Multicenter Automatic Defibrillator Implantation Trial-Cardiac Resynchronization Therapy). J Am Coll Cardiol. 2011;57(24):2416–23. PMID: 21658562.

41. Adabag S, Patton KK, Buxton AE, Rector TS, Ensrud KE, Vakil K, Levy WC, Poole JE. Association of implantable cardioverter defibrillators with survival in patients with and without improved ejection fraction: secondary analysis of the sudden cardiac death in heart failure trial. JAMA Cardiol. 2017;2(7):767–74. PMID: 28724134.

42. Moss AJ, Schuger C, Beck CA, Brown MW, Cannom DS, Daubert JP, Estes NA 3rd, Greenberg H, Hall WJ, Huang DT, Kautzner J, Klein H, McNitt S, Olshansky B, Shoda M, Wilber D, Zareba W, MADIT-RIT Trial Investigators. Reduction in inappropriate therapy and mortality through ICD programming. N Engl J Med. 2012;367(24):2275–83. PMID: 23131066.

43. Manne M, Rickard J, Varma N, Chung MK, Tchou P. Normalization of left ventricular ejection fraction after cardiac resynchronization therapy also normalizes survival. Pacing Clin Electrophysiol. 2013;36(8):970–7. PMID: 23718783.

44. Adabag AS, Therneau TM, Gersh BJ, Weston SA, Roger VL. Sudden death after myocardial infarction. JAMA. 2008;300(17):2022–9. PMID: 18984889.

45. Adabag AS, Maron BJ, Appelbaum E, Harrigan CJ, Buros JL, Gibson CM, Lesser JR, Hanna CA, Udelson JE, Manning WJ, Maron MS. Occurrence and frequency of arrhythmias in hypertrophic cardiomyopathy in relation to delayed enhancement on cardiovascular magnetic resonance. J Am Coll Cardiol. 2008;51(14):1369–74. PMID: 18387438.

46. Adabag S, Rector TS, Anand IS, McMurray JJ, Zile M, Komajda M, McKelvie RS, Massie B, Carson PE. A prediction model for sudden cardiac death in patients with heart failure and preserved ejection fraction. Eur J Heart Fail. 2014;16(11):1175–82. PMID: 25302657.

47. Adabag AS, Maron BJ. Implications of arrhythmias and prevention of sudden death in hypertrophic cardiomyopathy. Ann Noninvasive Electrocardiol. 2007;12(2):171–80. PMID: 17593187.

48. Al Aloul B, Adabag AS, Houghland MA, Tholakanahalli V. Brugada pattern electrocardiogram associated with supratherapeutic phenytoin levels and the risk of sudden death. Pacing Clin Electrophysiol. 2007;30(5):713–5. PMID: 17461883.

49. Gulati A, Jabbour A, Ismail TF, Guha K, Khwaja J, Raza S, Morarji K, Brown TD, Ismail NA, Dweck MR, Di Pietro E, Roughton M, Wage R, Daryani Y, O'Hanlon R, Sheppard MN, Alpendurada F, Lyon AR, Cook SA, Cowie MR, Assomull RG, Pennell DJ, Prasad SK. Association of fibrosis with mortality and sudden cardiac death in patients with nonischemic dilated cardiomyopathy. JAMA. 2013;309(9):896–908. PMID: 23462786.

50. Adabag AS, Luepker RV, Roger VL, Gersh BJ. Sudden cardiac death: epidemiology and risk factors. Nat Rev Cardiol. 2010;7(4):216–25. Epub 2010 Feb 9. PMID: 20142817.

51. Bardy GH, Lee KL, Mark DB, Poole JE, Packer DL, Boineau R, Domanski M, Troutman C, Anderson J, Johnson G, McNulty SE, Clapp-Channing N, Davidson-Ray LD, Fraulo ES, Fishbein DP, Luceri RM, Ip JH, Sudden Cardiac Death in Heart Failure Trial (SCD-HeFT) Investigators. Amiodarone or an implantable cardioverter-defibrillator for congestive heart failure. N Engl J Med. 2005;352(3):225–37. PMID: 15659722.

52. van Welsenes GH, van Rees JB, Borleffs CJ, Cannegieter SC, Bax JJ, van Erven L, Schalij MJ. Long-term follow-up of primary and secondary prevention implantable cardioverter defibrillator patients. Europace. 2011;13(3):389–94. Epub 2011 Jan 5. PMID: 21208947.
53. Køber L, Thune JJ, Nielsen JC, Haarbo J, Videbæk L, Korup E, Jensen G, Hildebrandt P, Steffensen FH, Bruun NE, Eiskjær H, Brandes A, Thøgersen AM, Gustafsson F, Egstrup K, Videbæk R, Hassager C, Svendsen JH, Høfsten DE, Torp-Pedersen C, Pehrson S, DANISH Investigators. Defibrillator implantation in patients with nonischemic systolic heart failure. N Engl J Med. 2016;375(13):1221–30. PMID: 27571011.
54. Anantha Narayanan M, Vakil K, Reddy YN, Baskaran J, Deshmukh A, Benditt DG, Adabag S. Efficacy of implantable cardioverter-defibrillator therapy in patients with nonischemic cardiomyopathy: a systematic review and meta-analysis of randomized controlled trials. JACC Clin Electrophysiol. 2017;3(9):962–70. PMID: 29759721.
55. Adabag S, Vo TN, Langsetmo L, Schousboe JT, Cawthon PM, Stone KL, Shikany JM, Taylor BC, Ensrud KE. Frailty as a risk factor for cardiovascular versus noncardiovascular mortality in older men: results from the MrOS sleep (outcomes of sleep disorders in older men) study. J Am Heart Assoc. 2018; 7(10): e008974.
56. Garcia S, Ko B, Adabag S. Contrast-induced nephropathy and risk of acute kidney injury and mortality after cardiac operations. Ann Thorac Surg. 2012;94(3):772–6. PMID: 22835553.
57. Buxton AE, Lee KL, Hafley GE, Pires LA, Fisher JD, Gold MR, Josephson ME, Lehmann MH, Prystowsky EN, MUSTT Investigators. Limitations of ejection fraction for prediction of sudden death risk in patients with coronary artery disease: lessons from the MUSTT study. J Am Coll Cardiol. 2007;50(12):1150–7. PMID: 17868806.
58. Coumbe AG, Naksuk N, Newell MC, Somasundaram PE, Benditt DG, Adabag S. Long-term follow-up of older patients with Mobitz type I second degree atrioventricular block. Heart. 2013;99(5):334–8. PMID: 23086974.
59. Moulki N, Kealhofer JV, Benditt DG, Gravely A, Vakil K, Garcia S, Adabag S. Association of cardiac implantable electronic devices with survival in bifascicular block prolonged PR interval on electrocardiogram. J Interv Card Electrophysiol. 2018;52:335–41. Epub ahead of print PMID: 29907894.

Chapter 9
Use of Implantable Monitors for Arrhythmia Detection

Jakub Tomala and Christopher Piorkowski

Introduction

Ambulatory ECG monitoring permits evaluation of transient cardiac electrical phenomena of brief duration over variable period of time. The initial recommendation included only two major indications: unexplained syncope, near syncope, or episodic dizziness and unexplained recurrent palpitations [1]. The indication spectrum of ambulatory ECG expanded vastly ever since.

The collected electrocardiographic data must be correlated to simultaneous occurrence of clinical symptoms. The recordings without this correlation are unlikely to establish their causative relationship. Only a minority of the patients (2–15%) will have an associated causal arrhythmia detected on a 24-h ECG monitoring [2]. Extending the time of recording significantly increases the likelihood of making the correct diagnosis [3, 4]. Consequently, the clinical need for prolonged ECG monitoring arose.

Implantable loop recorders (ILRs) are subcutaneous devices designed for ECG monitoring over a recording period of several years. This way, ILR can be very effective in finding a diagnosis in patients with very infrequent or asymptomatic episodes. Since their introduction in the 1990s [5], ILRs have played an increasing clinical role in the detection of cardiac arrhythmias.

The latest development regarding the device miniaturization as well as proprietary arrhythmia detection algorithms allowed this technology to be currently used in various clinical scenarios. Some of these are already reflected in recent national and international guidelines. Other newer indications for the continuous rhythm monitoring are still under evaluation and need to show an additional clinical benefit.

J. Tomala (✉) · C. Piorkowski
Heart Center Dresden University Hospital, Department of Invasive Electrophysiology, Dresden, Germany
e-mail: jakub.tomala@herzzentrum-dresden.com;
christopher.piorkowski@herzzentrum-dresden.com

© Springer Nature Switzerland AG 2019
J. S. Steinberg, A. E. Epstein (eds.), *Clinical Controversies in Device Therapy for Cardiac Arrhythmias*, https://doi.org/10.1007/978-3-030-22882-8_9

Evolution of Technology

Since their clinical introduction, ILRs have undergone an extensive process of technological development. Initially designed to store ECG recordings for temporal correlation between clinical symptoms and the actual cardiac rhythm, ILRs have been later equipped with automatic algorithms in order to monitor occurrence and burden of cardiac arrhythmias independently from the symptoms. The Reveal XT was the first representative of this ILR generation, designed for automatic detection of atrial fibrillation (AF) [6]. Limited detection performance with a high amount of false-positive episodes resulted in overall positive predictive values of about 30% for all automatically recorded AF episodes [7] with little clinical use.

It was only recently that developments of the latest ILR generation (Reveal LINQ) have improved automatic AF detection algorithms to a nearly 100% sensitivity and positive predictive values close to 90% [8]. This was a crucial step for automated arrhythmia assessment and related advances in clinical patient management in the upcoming years.

Furthermore, ILRs have been miniaturized to a level when they can be subcutaneously injected rather than surgically implanted.

ILRs are nowadays equipped with remote monitoring functionalities accessible through large telemedicine network coverage.

Established Fields of Indications

Palpitations

ILR readily detects arrhythmias associated with palpitations. However, upon exclusion of structural heart disease, such arrhythmias only seldom confer malignant prognosis [9, 10]. Thus the diagnostic process in this setting is primarily driven by patient symptoms. The more frequent the symptoms get, the higher is the probability of detecting the causative arrhythmia with other means of ambulatory ECG monitoring (Holter monitor or event monitor). It has been shown that patients with recurrent palpitations benefit from an electrophysiology study without having to record the actual clinical tachycardia [11]. Albeit ILRs have proven to be effective [12], their role in this patient collective appears limited to those with inconclusive initial diagnostic workup and persistent symptoms. In such cases the differentiation between cardiac and noncardiac etiology can help reduce otherwise frequent unscheduled visits to the emergency department [13] and potentially improve the quality of life.

Syncope

Patients presenting with syncope exhibit a wide spectrum of underlying etiologies. Based on the known prognostic implications, the identification of those with cardiac syncope remains crucial [14]. The widely used tilt testing has a low diagnostic yield in patients with likely vasovagal syncope as well as it lacks the desired negative predictive value [15, 16]. Therefore, the role of prolonged ECG monitoring became even more emphasized. There is compelling evidence that ILRs significantly increase the diagnostic rate in unselected syncopal patients and allow an ECG-directed treatment with reduction in syncopal events and improved quality of life [17]. This has been further highlighted in various clinically challenging subpopulations, such as patients with negative workup and bundle branch block, older patients, and patients with unexplained falls [18–20]. Besides the identification of the culprit arrhythmia in cardiac syncope, there are potential benefits for patients with reflex syncope. Although pacing in reflex syncope remains a controversial strategy, ILRs could prove useful in determining whether the patients with suspected cardioinhibitory response would benefit from a pacemaker [21]. In certain cases, the scope of diagnostic use of ILR even exceeds cardiac arrhythmias. Monitoring with ILR showed a high rate of misdiagnosis of epilepsy [22]. This finding advocates the use of prolonged ECG monitoring in patients with unsatisfactory response to therapy with anticonvulsant medication. Additionally, a number of patients with generalized tonic-clonic seizures had a specific myopotential pattern recognized on the ECG tracings [23]. There is sufficient evidence that ILR should be employed early in the diagnostic process of syncopal patients leading to reduced recurrence rate and improved quality of life [24, 25] and could help reduce the overall costs [26]. The role of remote monitoring and necessary length of the monitoring in this setting is still a matter of discussion. However, there is data showing that cumulative diagnostic rates continue to increase up to 4 years after the implantation [27].

Evolving Fields of Indications

Atrial Fibrillation

AF monitoring is a new and evolving field of ILR usage. ILR-based AF detection is primarily derived from the characteristic incoherence in the RR intervals over a certain period of time. Though implantable devices with atrial leads are considered as the gold standard for continuous long-term AF detection [28], ILRs have been shown to have a high sensitivity (>98%) [6] and excellent positive predictive value [8] in detecting AF episodes. The diagnosis of AF encompasses diverse patient groups requiring different therapeutic approaches.

Clinical Management

Clinical AF management centers around two fundamental pillars. One relates to the decision for rhythm or rate control. The other deals with the indication for oral anticoagulants (OAC).

In patients with a pure rate control strategy is any sophisticated monitoring tool less likely to be needed. The 24-h ECG Holter is an effective measure to ascertain the ventricular response rate during active and rest periods of the day. That changes in patients in whom rhythm control becomes the treatment of choice. AF pattern, AF burden, and the presence of other coexisting brady- or tachyarrhythmias influence the overall clinical management. The indications for catheter ablation, further cardiac device therapy, antiarrhythmic medication, assessment of their efficacy, and side effects control are likely to be affected by ILR monitoring. In that respect comes the patient with AF and heart failure into the center of attention. The AF burden that drives patients into heart failure may become an important parameter for clinical decision-making. In addition, continuous ILR monitoring provides the ability of ventricular arrhythmia detection and stratification of the sudden cardiac death (SCD) risk of this specific patient cohort. In a trial of hypertensive patients with signs of left ventricular hypertrophy, even a new-onset AF itself showed to be a significant predictor of SCD [29].

Regarding the indications for OAC in current medical practice, ECG monitoring seems to be of lesser relevance. They are primarily based on estimated stroke risk derived from several clinical risk factors, as presented in the $CHADS_2$ and CHA_2DS_2-VASc score. However, these composite risk scores have been derived from cohorts predominantly made up of patients suffering from persistent or permanent AF [30, 31]. It remains debatable whether patients with paroxysmal AF and a much lower AF burden suffer from the same stroke risk. This question can only be addressed with help of continuous monitoring data from devices such as ILR. Subsequently, continuous monitoring may have a role in decision-making on OAC in clinical routine.

Post-ablation Monitoring

The quality of monitoring after catheter ablation of AF is an everlasting topic. Post-ablation outcome assessment is challenged by (i) asymptomatic recurrences, (ii) short episodes, (iii) various follow-up duration due to re-ablation timing, and (iv) individual healing duration and post-ablation recurrence patterns [32]. Success rates of AF ablation remain controversial, since many previous studies are based on symptom-reporting and intermittent ECG monitoring, which underestimate the actual recurrence rates. From a clinical perspective, it is essential to rely upon appropriate detection of AF to make decisions concerning antiarrhythmic therapy. Moreover, reliable diagnosis of AF is scientifically warranted when evaluating new therapeutic approaches. Therefore, ILRs are being increasingly used in patients who underwent catheter ablation of AF. Distinct post-ablation rhythm profiles with potential links to pathophysiology and arrhythmia mechanism have been described in a recent registry [8]. The assessment of AF burden and detection of prolonged healing phases could unfold the potential of ILRs in individualized patient care.

Besides arrhythmia control, the role of ILRs also extends into the topic of OAC. In a number of retrospective registries, low rates of stroke were generally observed in patients after catheter ablation [33, 34]. As randomized trial data is still lacking, it is unclear if a successful catheter ablation reduces the risk of stroke and hence justifies discontinuation of OAC in selected patients. An ongoing trial has been designed to investigate the option of recurrence-guided intermittent OAC based on ILR recordings in patients with moderate risk of thromboembolism [35]. In spite of this appealing strategy, the stroke risk in AF patients is not only linked to the presence or absence of AF as cases of thromboembolic stroke in recurrence-free patients have been described. Therefore, a more complex and individualized approach combining detection of AF together with additional, nonconventional risk factors such as atrial transport function may prove helpful in tackling this challenge. Other potential indications for post-interventional continuous rhythm monitoring include patients after ablation of typical atrial flutter, patients after surgical ablation procedures, and possibly patients after other cardiac surgery.

Cryptogenic Stroke

AF detection in patients with cryptogenic stroke could become the first clinical scenario in which the use of ILR shows outcome-relevant scientific evidence of superiority over standard intermittent Holter monitoring. After a follow-up of 3 years, the AF detection rate with ILR reached 30%. ILR was able to detect ten times more patients with mostly asymptomatic AF as compared to intermittent Holter recording [36, 37]. All of these patients have already experienced one of the most debilitating complications of AF – a stroke. The immediate clinical consequence of the diagnosis, initiation of OAC, is expected to significantly reduce the rate of recurrent thromboembolism.

The strategy of initiating OAC in patients with cryptogenic stroke by default, i.e., without the confirmed diagnosis of AF or an identified cardioembolic source, has been explored in a respective trial. However, this attempt to avoid continuous ECG monitoring failed to demonstrate superiority over the standard treatment and was associated with a higher risk of bleeding [38]. This finding shifts the clinical focus back toward continuous ECG monitoring as a means to identify the patients who will benefit from OAC.

In the future, it will be desirable to monitor high-risk populations in order to prevent strokes upfront. That would enhance the use of ILR as a diagnostic tool for both secondary and primary stroke prevention. The respective studies are ongoing [39].

Risk Stratification and Sudden Cardiac Death

Cardiac arrhythmias exhibit a great variability not only in their symptoms but also in their prognostic value. These depend on the specific clinical presentation and the underlying condition. ILR demonstrated sufficient sensitivity to detect ventricular tachycardia (VT) and ventricular fibrillation (VF) [40] and could prove useful in risk stratification of patients with, or predisposed to, malignant arrhythmias and SCD.

Myocardial Infarction and Ischemic Heart Disease

Myocardial infarction (MI) confers a transient risk of SCD due to arrhythmias associated with acute ischemia. In addition, there is a long-term risk of reentry tachycardia at the borders of a ventricular scar. The occurrence of non-sustained ventricular tachycardia (NSVT) has been proposed as a potential risk factor for subsequent malignant tachyarrhythmias and SCD. So far, clinical trials using intermittent and continuous monitoring presented conflicting evidence on this topic [41–44]. Therefore, the concept of continuous rhythm monitoring with ILR in post-MI patients with LVEF >35% is being currently revisited. The BIOGUARD-MI study pairs ILR monitoring with standardized and early telemedicine-triggered clinical interventions [39].

Cardiomyopathies

In contrast to ischemic cardiomyopathy, the mechanisms of arrhythmogenesis in nonischemic dilated cardiomyopathy (DCM) are more variable. The occurring ventricular arrhythmias may be related to structural changes such as fibrosis and left ventricular dilation as well as to primary and secondary electrophysiological changes. Although current guidelines for primary prevention in patients with DCM rely on LVEF and functional class, these parameters are neither specific nor sensitive enough to identify the patients with highest risk of SCD. Many SCDs occur in patients with LVEF >35% and many patients with LVEF<35% die of other causes [45]. Therefore, other predictors of adverse outcome have been proposed. Such predictors include microvolt T-wave alternans, signal-averaged-ECG, QRS duration, fragmented QRS, QRS-T angle, and NSVT [46]. Whether the employment of ILR in assessment of these parameters is of added value remains an interesting question to be addressed in the future.

Although the risk of SCD in hypertrophic cardiomyopathy remains relatively low [47], the occurrence of NSVT has been shown to be the most important factor in its prediction [48]. ILR has been already employed in monitoring of patients after the alcohol septal ablation [49], but its clinical role in overall risk stratification of SCD has yet to be established.

Infiltrative cardiomyopathies, such as amyloidosis, sarcoidosis, and Fabry disease, are well correlated with ventricular arrhythmias and SCD. The use of ILR in these patients showed that clinically relevant arrhythmias are often missed with intermittent ECG monitoring [50]. It has been further demonstrated that the harbinger of terminal cardiac decompensation is often bradycardia [51].

In patients with tachycardia-induced cardiomyopathy, the decline in LVEF develops slowly over time and appears reversible. However, repetitive tachycardia relapses cause rapid deterioration of systolic function and development of progressive heart failure [52]. Understandably, continuous rhythm monitoring appears to be crucial in this setting. Trials designed to investigate specific risk factors, effects of rhythm restoration [53], as well as the impact of ILR monitoring on overall heart failure management [54] are ongoing.

Inherited Arrhythmia Syndromes and Congenital Heart Disease

There is evidence that the use of ILR in patients with primary arrhythmia syndromes may be useful for therapy guidance. As the majority of symptoms represent benign rhythms, they play a role in reassuring patients and physicians that no further intervention is required in some cases [55].

The evidence for monitoring with ILR in congenital heart disease is rather anecdotal. Nevertheless, given its purely diagnostic character and excellent safety profile, ILR may represent a viable option for patients who do not qualify for the implantation of an ICD.

ILR Versus Wearable Technologies

Apart from the recent evolution of ILRs, other methods of rhythm monitoring have undergone a substantial development as well. These are mostly based on surface ECG electrodes (patches and event monitors) or photoplethysmography (heart rate monitors, wristwatches). Although such devices compete with ILR as a screening tool for larger populations [56], it is questionable whether they can become a relevant alternative in clinical patient management. Irrespective of their accuracy and detection algorithms, these wearables still provide only intermittent monitoring.

References

1. Crawford MH, Bernstein SJ, Deedwania PC, et al. ACC/AHA guidelines for ambulatory electrocardiography: a report of the American College of Cardiology/American Heart Association Task Force on practice guidelines (Committee to Revise the Guidelines for Ambulatory Electrocardiography) developed in collaboration with the North American Society for Pacing and Electrophysiology. J Am Coll Cardiol. 1999;34:912–48.
2. Zeldis SM, Levine BJ, Michelson EL, Morganroth J. Cardiovascular complaints. Correlation with cardiac arrhythmias on 24-hour electrocardiographic monitoring. Chest. 1980;78:456–61.
3. Gibson TC, Heitzman MR. Diagnostic efficacy of 24-hour electrocardiographic monitoring for syncope. Am J Cardiol. 1984;53:1013–7.

4. Bass EB, Curtiss EI, Arena VC, Hanusa BH, Cecchetti A, Karpf M, Kapoor WN. The duration of Holter monitoring in patients with syncope. Is 24 hours enough? Arch Intern Med. 1990;150:1073–8.
5. Krahn AD, Klein GJ, Yee R, Norris C. Final results from a pilot study with an implantable loop recorder to determine the etiology of syncope in patients with negative noninvasive and invasive testing. Am J Cardiol. 1998;82:117–9.
6. Hindricks G, Pokushalov E, Urban L, Taborsky M, Kuck K-H, Lebedev D, Rieger G, Pürerfellner H, XPECT Trial Investigators. Performance of a new leadless implantable cardiac monitor in detecting and quantifying atrial fibrillation: results of the XPECT trial. Circ Arrhythm Electrophysiol. 2010;3:141–7.
7. Eitel C, Husser D, Hindricks G, Frühauf M, Hilbert S, Arya A, Gaspar T, Wetzel U, Bollmann A, Piorkowski C. Performance of an implantable automatic atrial fibrillation detection device: impact of software adjustments and relevance of manual episode analysis. Europace. 2011;13:480–5.
8. Wechselberger S, Kronborg M, Huo Y, et al. Continuous monitoring after atrial fibrillation ablation: the LINQ AF study. EP Eur. 2018;20:f312–20.
9. Knudson MP. The natural history of palpitations in a family practice. J Fam Pract. 1987;24:357–60.
10. Weber BE, Kapoor WN. Evaluation and outcomes of patients with palpitations. Am J Med. 1996;100:138–48.
11. Lauschke J, Schneider J, Schneider R, Nesselmann C, Tischer T, Glass A, Bänsch D. Electrophysiological studies in patients with paroxysmal supraventricular tachycardias but no electrocardiogram documentation: findings from a prospective registry. Europace. 2015;17:801–6.
12. Giada F, Gulizia M, Francese M, Croci F, Santangelo L, Santomauro M, Occhetta E, Menozzi C, Raviele A. Recurrent unexplained palpitations (RUP) study comparison of implantable loop recorder versus conventional diagnostic strategy. J Am Coll Cardiol. 2007;49:1951–6.
13. Kroenke K, Arrington ME, Mangelsdorff AD. The prevalence of symptoms in medical outpatients and the adequacy of therapy. Arch Intern Med. 1990;150:1685–9.
14. Soteriades ES, Evans JC, Larson MG, Chen MH, Chen L, Benjamin EJ, Levy D. Incidence and prognosis of syncope. N Engl J Med. 2002;347:878–85.
15. Deharo J-C, Jego C, Lanteaume A, Djiane P. An implantable loop recorder study of highly symptomatic vasovagal patients. J Am Coll Cardiol. 2006;47:587–93.
16. Brignole M, Sutton R, Menozzi C, et al. Lack of correlation between the responses to tilt testing and adenosine triphosphate test and the mechanism of spontaneous neurally mediated syncope. Eur Heart J. 2006;27:2232–9.
17. Farwell DJ, Freemantle N, Sulke N. The clinical impact of implantable loop recorders in patients with syncope. Eur Heart J. 2006;27:351–6.
18. Da Costa A, Defaye P, Romeyer-Bouchard C, et al. Clinical impact of the implantable loop recorder in patients with isolated syncope, bundle branch block and negative workup: a randomized multicentre prospective study. Arch Cardiovasc Dis. 2013;106:146–54.
19. Armstrong VL, Lawson J, Kamper AM, Newton J, Kenny RA. The use of an implantable loop recorder in the investigation of unexplained syncope in older people. Age Ageing. 2003;32:185–8.
20. Bhangu J, McMahon CG, Hall P, Bennett K, Rice C, Crean P, Sutton R, Kenny R-A. Long-term cardiac monitoring in older adults with unexplained falls and syncope. Heart. 2016;102:681–6.
21. Brignole M, Deharo JC, Menozzi C, Moya A, Sutton R, Tomaino M, Ungar A. The benefit of pacemaker therapy in patients with neurally mediated syncope and documented asystole: a meta-analysis of implantable loop recorder studies. Europace. 2017;20:1362–6.
22. Petkar S, Hamid T, Iddon P, Clifford A, Rice N, Claire R, McKee D, Curtis N, Cooper PN, Fitzpatrick AP. Prolonged implantable electrocardiographic monitoring indicates a high rate of misdiagnosis of epilepsy – REVISE study. Europace. 2012;14:1653–60.
23. Ho RT, Wicks T, Wyeth D, Nei M. Generalized tonic-clonic seizures detected by implantable loop recorder devices: diagnosing more than cardiac arrhythmias. Heart Rhythm. 2006;3:857–61.

24. Podoleanu C, DaCosta A, Defaye P, et al. Early use of an implantable loop recorder in syncope evaluation: a randomized study in the context of the French healthcare system (FRESH study). Arch Cardiovasc Dis. 2014;107:546–52.
25. Sulke N, Sugihara C, Hong P, Patel N, Freemantle N. The benefit of a remotely monitored implantable loop recorder as a first line investigation in unexplained syncope: the EaSyAS II trial. Europace. 2016;18:912–8.
26. Edvardsson N, Wolff C, Tsintzos S, Rieger G, Linker NJ. Costs of unstructured investigation of unexplained syncope: insights from a micro-costing analysis of the observational PICTURE registry. Europace. 2015;17:1141–8.
27. Furukawa T, Maggi R, Bertolone C, Fontana D, Brignole M. Additional diagnostic value of very prolonged observation by implantable loop recorder in patients with unexplained syncope. J Cardiovasc Electrophysiol. 2012;23:67–71.
28. Purerfellner H, Gillis AM, Holbrook R, Hettrick DA. Accuracy of atrial tachyarrhythmia detection in implantable devices with arrhythmia therapies. Pacing Clin Electrophysiol. 2004;27:983–92.
29. Okin PM, Bang CN, Wachtell K, Hille DA, Kjeldsen SE, Dahlöf B, Devereux RB. Relationship of sudden cardiac death to new-onset atrial fibrillation in hypertensive patients with left ventricular hypertrophy. Circ Arrhythmia Electrophysiol. 2013;6:243–51.
30. Gage BF, Waterman AD, Shannon W, Boechler M, Rich MW, Radford MJ. Validation of clinical classification schemes for predicting stroke: results from the National Registry of Atrial Fibrillation. JAMA. 2001;285:2864–70.
31. Lip GYH, Nieuwlaat R, Pisters R, Lane DA, Crijns HJGM. Refining clinical risk stratification for predicting stroke and thromboembolism in atrial fibrillation using a novel risk factor-based approach: the euro heart survey on atrial fibrillation. Chest. 2010;137:263–72.
32. Hindricks G, Piorkowski C, Tanner H, Kobza R, Gerds-Li J-H, Carbucicchio C, Kottkamp H. Perception of atrial fibrillation before and after radiofrequency catheter ablation: relevance of asymptomatic arrhythmia recurrence. Circulation. 2005;112:307–13.
33. Karasoy D, Gislason GH, Hansen J, Johannessen A, Køber L, Hvidtfeldt M, Özcan C, Torp-Pedersen C, Hansen ML. Oral anticoagulation therapy after radiofrequency ablation of atrial fibrillation and the risk of thromboembolism and serious bleeding: long-term follow-up in nationwide cohort of Denmark. Eur Heart J. 2015;36:307–14a.
34. Ha ACT, Hindricks G, Birnie DH, Verma A. Long-term oral anticoagulation for patients after successful catheter ablation of atrial fibrillation. Curr Opin Cardiol. 2015;30:1–7.
35. Passman R, Leong-Sit P, Andrei A-C, Huskin A, Tomson TT, Bernstein R, Ellis E, Waks JW, Zimetbaum P. Targeted anticoagulation for atrial fibrillation guided by continuous rhythm assessment with an insertable cardiac monitor: the rhythm evaluation for anticoagulation with continuous monitoring (REACT.COM) pilot study. J Cardiovasc Electrophysiol. 2016;27:264–70.
36. Sanna T, Diener H-C, Passman RS, et al. Cryptogenic stroke and underlying atrial fibrillation. N Engl J Med. 2014;370:2478–86.
37. Thijs VN, Brachmann J, Morillo CA, et al. Predictors for atrial fibrillation detection after cryptogenic stroke: results from CRYSTAL AF. Neurology. 2016;86:261–9.
38. Hart RG, Sharma M, Mundl H, et al. Rivaroxaban for stroke prevention after embolic stroke of undetermined source. N Engl J Med. 2018;378:2191–201.
39. BIO monitorinG in patients with preserved left ventricular function after diagnosed myocardial infarction (BIOlGUARD-MI). ClinicalTrials.gov [Internet]. Bethesda: National Library of Medicine (US). 2015. Identifier NCT02341534, Available from: http://clinicaltrials.gov/ct2/show/study/NCT02341534.
40. Volosin K, Stadler RW, Wyszynski R, Kirchhof P. Tachycardia detection performance of implantable loop recorders: results from a large "real-life" patient cohort and patients with induced ventricular arrhythmias. Europace. 2013;15:1215–22.
41. Bloch Thomsen PE, Jons C, Raatikainen MJP, et al. Long-term recording of cardiac arrhythmias with an implantable cardiac monitor in patients with reduced ejection fraction after acute myocardial Infarction. Circulation. 2010;122:1258–64.

42. La Rovere MT, Pinna GD, Hohnloser SH, Marcus FI, Mortara A, Nohara R, Bigger JT, Camm AJ, Schwartz PJ, ATRAMI Investigators. Autonomic tone and reflexes after myocardial infarction. Baroreflex sensitivity and heart rate variability in the identification of patients at risk for life-threatening arrhythmias: implications for clinical trials. Circulation. 2001;103:2072–7.
43. Scirica BM, Braunwald E, Belardinelli L, Hedgepeth CM, Spinar J, Wang W, Qin J, Karwatowska-Prokopczuk E, Verheugt FWA, Morrow DA. Relationship between nonsustained ventricular tachycardia after non–ST-elevation acute coronary syndrome and sudden cardiac death. Circulation. 2010;122:455–62.
44. Piccini JP, White JA, Mehta RH, et al. Sustained ventricular tachycardia and ventricular fibrillation complicating non–ST-segment–elevation acute coronary syndromes. Circulation. 2012;126:41–9.
45. Hohnloser SH, Kuck KH, Dorian P, Roberts RS, Hampton JR, Hatala R, Fain E, Gent M, Connolly SJ, DINAMIT Investigators. Prophylactic use of an implantable cardioverter–defibrillator after acute myocardial Infarction. N Engl J Med. 2004;351:2481–8.
46. Goldberger JJ, Subačius H, Patel T, Cunnane R, Kadish AH. Sudden cardiac death risk stratification in patients with nonischemic dilated cardiomyopathy. J Am Coll Cardiol. 2014;63:1879–89.
47. Veselka J, Faber L, Liebregts M, et al. Outcome of alcohol septal ablation in mildly symptomatic patients with hypertrophic obstructive cardiomyopathy: a long-term follow-up study based on the euro-alcohol septal ablation registry. J Am Heart Assoc. 2017;6:e005735.
48. O'Mahony C, Jichi F, Pavlou M, et al. A novel clinical risk prediction model for sudden cardiac death in hypertrophic cardiomyopathy (HCM risk-SCD). Eur Heart J. 2014;35:2010–20.
49. Balt JC, Wijffels MCEF, Boersma LVA, Wever EFD, ten Berg JM. Continuous rhythm monitoring for ventricular arrhythmias after alcohol septal ablation for hypertrophic cardiomyopathy. Heart. 2014;100:1865–70.
50. Weidemann F, Maier SKG, Störk S, et al. Usefulness of an implantable loop recorder to detect clinically relevant arrhythmias in patients with advanced Fabry cardiomyopathy. Am J Cardiol. 2016;118:264–74.
51. Sayed RH, Rogers D, Khan F, et al. A study of implanted cardiac rhythm recorders in advanced cardiac AL amyloidosis. Eur Heart J. 2015;36:1098–105.
52. Nerheim P, Birger-Botkin S, Piracha L, Olshansky B. Heart failure and sudden death in patients with tachycardia-induced cardiomyopathy and recurrent tachycardia. Circulation. 2004;110:247–52.
53. Risk Factors in Tachycardiomyopathy (EMPATHY). ClinicalTrials.gov [Internet]. Bethesda: National Library of Medicine (US); 2018. Identifier NCT03418467, Available from: http://clinicaltrials.gov/ct2/show/study/NCT03418467.
54. Reveal LINQ™ Heart Failure (LINQ HF). ClinicalTrials.gov [Internet]. Bethesda: National Library of Medicine (US); 2016. Identifier NCT02758301, Available from: http://clinicaltrials.gov/ct2/show/study/NCT02758301.
55. Avari Silva JN, Bromberg BI, Emge FK, Bowman TM, Van Hare GF. Implantable loop recorder monitoring for refining management of children with inherited arrhythmia syndromes. J Am Heart Assoc. 2016;5:e003632.
56. Apple Heart Study: Assessment of Wristwatch-Based Photoplethysmography to Identify Cardiac Arrhythmias. ClinicalTrials.gov [Internet]. Bethesda: National Library of Medicine (US); 2017. Identifier NCT03335800, Available from: http://clinicaltrials.gov/ct2/show/NCT03335800.

Chapter 10
Ethical Conundra in CIED Therapy: Ethical Implantation, Ethical End-of-Life Care

Rachel Lampert

Implantable cardioverter-defibrillators save lives in multiple populations of patients at risk for life-threatening ventricular arrhythmias, as described in prior chapters. However, ICD shocks are painful, described by patients as "being kicked by a mule" or "putting a finger in a light socket" [1], decreasing quality of life [2]. For a patient who otherwise has many years of quality life left, survival from cardiac arrest may be worth the trade-off of painful shocks. However, for those with life-limiting illnesses, shocks may create pain without meaningfully increasing lifespan. For patients with a previously implanted ICD now nearing the end of life, ethical patient care demands ongoing discussions of goals of care and how the options of continuing shocking function versus deactivation of the ICD may fit with current goals. Dying peacefully is valued by all – as described by relatives, peaceful death is an indicator of quality in palliative care [3].

For patients with apparent indications for ICD based on purely cardiac risk factors for sudden death [4, 5], ethical patient care demands holistic understanding of benefit of the ICD, as well as of patient goals and preferences. Implantation of an ICD in a patient with minimal chance of significant prolongation of life not only exposes the patient to risks of the procedure but to painful shocks.

Relationships with industry: Dr Lampert has received significant research funding from Boston Scientific, Medtronic, and Abbott/St Jude Medical (significant),and has received honoraria and consulting fees from Medtronic (modest).

R. Lampert (✉)
Yale University School of Medicine, New Haven, CT, USA
e-mail: rachel.lampert@yale.edu

© Springer Nature Switzerland AG 2019
J. S. Steinberg, A. E. Epstein (eds.), *Clinical Controversies in Device Therapy for Cardiac Arrhythmias*, https://doi.org/10.1007/978-3-030-22882-8_10

Ethical Implantation

Benefit and Comorbidities

Indications for defibrillator implantation for primary prevention, based on landmark trials showing benefit in patients with decreased ejection fraction and congestive heart failure and/or myocardial infarction, are well-known, and recent guidelines have changed little since 2008 [4, 5]. However, perhaps less widely known is the first class III indication in the guidelines, "ICD therapy is not indicated for patients who do not have a reasonable expectation of survival with an acceptable functional status for at least 1 year, even if they meet ICD implantation criteria specified in the class I, IIa, and IIb recommendations above *(Level of Evidence: C)*."[4] Palliative care experts are consulted not uncommonly regarding device activation in patients with recent implants [6], which has raised the question whether implanting electrophysiologists may ignore medical severe comorbidities that might limit the benefit of ICDs [6]. However, in one reported series [7] of patients requesting deactivation, the three patients in whom malignancy had been diagnosed prior to device implant had all been given greater-than-one-year life expectancies by their oncologist. The AMA Code of Ethics requires that physicians not impose on patients therapies which may be medically futile [8]. However, medical futility may be difficult to determine. A "reasonable expectation of survival for more than one year," a relatively "hard" endpoint, can already be difficult to predict in many cases; "reasonable expectation of survival with good functional status" even more difficult to define.

Two patient populations may require particular attention to comorbidities and expected functional status. To what extent ICDs benefit the elderly is an oft-raised question [9]. One editorialist has asked, "Is anyone too old for an implantable cardioverter-defibrillator" [10]? The median age in the landmark trials of ICD benefit has been in the 60s. While randomized trial data in the elderly are lacking, and results of meta-analyses variable [11, 12], other data do suggest benefit in the elderly. For example, while survival after ICD implantation is shorter in the elderly (as in any population), rates of appropriate device therapies are similar [13]. Two observational studies have suggested benefit in elderly—in a propensity-matched analysis of ICD patients in the Medicare population, the adjusted hazard ratio for mortality with an ICD was 0.62 [14], and in an analysis of the Get With The Guidelines population, HR was 0.71 [15]. In a subanalysis of the MADIT II trial, the subset of patients over age 75 years had greater benefit than younger patients [16]. In general, ICDs are less likely to decrease quality of life in the elderly than in the young [17].

However, it is clear that comorbidities play a critical role in survival benefit in this population. While age has minimal impact on surgical morbidity and mortality for device implantation, comorbidity significantly worsens procedural and in-hospital outcomes [18, 19]. In an analysis combining data from the National Cardiovascular Data Registry (NCDR) ICD Registry with Medicare data, 10% of ICD recipients met criteria for frailty, and those with this geriatric condition had a

1-year mortality twice that of those without; frailty in combination with other comorbidities such as COPD or diabetes synergistically increased mortality [20]. As comorbidities increase, ICD benefit decreases, particularly in the elderly [21].

Patients suffering from dementia represent another group in whom ethical care requires particular attention. As medicine continues to advance and life is increasingly prolonged, the number of patients going on to develop dementia is expected to increase from 35 million people worldwide currently to 115 million by 2050 [22]. One study combining data from the NCDR ICD Registry with Medicare data suggests that 1% of patients receiving a de novo ICD may suffer from dementia [20]. How ICDs impact quality of life in patients with dementia is unknown. Shocks increase catecholamines even in patients under deep sedation [23], and patients with dementia express pain through facial expression and changes in behavior [22].

Decision-making around de novo ICD implantation for those in the continuum from mild cognitive impairment to dementia requires careful discussion of risks and benefits in the context of patient values and preferences. Using data from the NDCR ICD Registry combined with Medicare, Green et al. found that 1% of those receiving de novo ICDs had dementia. Mortality in these patients was 27% at 1 year, similar to that in patients with solid tumors [20]. Mortality after a diagnosis of dementia in the general population is high, with an estimated median survival after onset of dementia of 1.3 [24] to 3.3 years [25], similar to that of more commonly recognized end-of-life conditions as metastatic breast cancer and stage IV congestive heart failure. Guidelines recommend against ICDs for patients in whom good functional status at 1 year is not expected [4], and many patients with advanced dementia will fall in that group. For individuals less severely impacted by dementia, shared decision-making around ICD implantation is crucial [26]. Ensuring that patients and families understand the risk of mortality after ICD implant, as well as the possibility of painful shocks, is critical to help patients and families think about ICD implant in the setting of the patient values and preferences. Proxies are less likely to choose aggressive interventions when they are aware of the poor prognosis carried by dementia [27]. However it may be particularly complicated to weigh the benefit/burden ratio of ICD implantation in patients with mild cognitive impairment or the earlier stages of dementia, because in general these patients have relatively maintained quality of life in the early stages, and as such patients and families may opt for decreasing the risk of sudden cardiac death.

Decision-Making Around ICD Implantation

For all patients, ethical device implantation requires a shared decision-making model as this option is discussed. Medicine has entered an era of patient-centered care, in which the paternalistic concept that doctors know best and should thus make decisions for their patients has been replaced by a model that fosters patient-clinician collaboration. Shared decision-making (SDM), termed the "pinnacle of patient-centered care," is the process by which clinicians and patients work together to develop care plans based on clinical evidence that balance risks and expected outcomes with patient preferences and values [26]. Making recommendations for an ICD without taking into account patients goals of care is inconsistent with medical ethical principles of autonomy [28]. For a patient with heart failure, the decision in considering an ICD is not between life and death but rather between accepting an ICD and having a potentially longer life with advancing heart failure or declining an ICD and having a potentially shorter life but maintaining the opportunity to die quickly [9]. Current heart failure guidelines specifically state that this trade-off should be discussed [29], and CMS now mandates a SDM interaction prior to CID implantation for patients prior to implantation of a device for primary prevention [30].

Data suggest that decision-making around ICD implantation is currently suboptimal. Multiple studies [31, 32], as recently as last year [33], show significant misunderstanding about risks and benefits of ICDs. One survey of physicians described that physicians avoided discussion of risks of ICD in order to steer the patient away from a "bad decision" [34]. Further, detailed interview studies of patients considering ICDs reveal multiple cognitive biases in both those who accept and those who decline the device, further complicating decision-making [32, 35]. Many patients report not being told of the option of not getting an ICD or not being asked whether they wanted the device [36].

The current CMS coverage decision mandates not just SDM, but use of an "evidence-based decision tool on ICDs" prior to implantation [30]. One example is found at https://patientdecisionaid.org/wp-content/uploads/2017/01/ICD-Infographic-5.23.16.pdf. In a recent Cochrane review [37] of 105 studies comparing use of decision-aids with general information for a variety of diseases, those using these tools felt better-informed with more accurate understanding of benefits and harms, as well as making decisions more consistent with their values. The tools did not worsen health outcomes and did not impact satisfaction. Early data evaluating the recommended tool for decision-making for primary prevention ICD implantation [38] suggested that it increased knowledge and satisfaction and reduced decisional conflict and regret. Further research is needed to determine whether widespread, mandated use of a decision-aid for patients undergoing ICD implantation will improve the decision-making process.

Ethical End of Life Care

For patients with an ICD implanted previously, ethical care as patients near the end of life mandates discussion of deactivation of the shocking function. The experience of dying patients receiving ICD shocks was first reported in the palliative care literature ("Death and Dying, a Shocking Experience" [39], "And It Can Go On and On and On…") [40]. Through interviewing families of recently deceased ICD patients, Goldstein et al. found that 20% reported that their family member received shocks in the last weeks, days, or hours of their lives [41]. This number was likely an underestimate; however, as in many cases, family may not have been aware of shocks received. More recently, Kinch Westerdahl et al. [42] definitively determined the frequency of shocks while dying, performing postmortem ICD interrogation in 130 consecutive patients. Close to one-third received a shock in their last 24 h, many of whom had storms of over ten shocks, experiencing unnecessary pain while dying.

To what extent the failure to deactivate therapies stems from patient choice versus failure of the physician to communicate this option is unknown. Studies of patient preferences regarding ICD deactivation at end of life have shown mixed results. Several written surveys of ICD patients regarding preferences for ICD deactivation in hypothetical situations have found that patients may not wish deactivation even in the setting of constant dyspnea or frequent shocks [43]. In the only series of patients actually facing the decision in whom the option of deactivation was discussed – six patients with terminal malignancies, all with a history of treated ventricular arrhythmias – none chose to turn off shocking therapies [7]. However, we found, in a recent interview study, again a survey of hypothetical situations, putting ICD deactivation in the context of health outcomes such as functional and cognitive disability known to influence decision-making, that most would at least hypothetically choose deactivation in some situations [44]. Thus it is more likely that the high number of patients who die with device therapies active does so not out of conscious choice but because they did not know deactivation was an option.

In order to decrease shocks and improve quality of life in dying patients, the Heart Rhythm Society convened a multidisciplinary group of doctors, nurses, patients, lawyers, and ethicists, whose recommendations were published in 2010 in the "HRS Expert Consensus Statement on the Management of Cardiovascular Implantable Electronic Devices (CIEDs) in patients nearing end of life or requesting withdrawal of therapy" [45]. This document described the ethical and legal underpinnings of deactivation of ICDs and highlighted the importance of proactive communication around ICD deactivation by clinicians.

Ethical and Legal Principles Underlying Deactivation

As discussed in detail in the HRS document, deactivation of ICDs at a patient's request is strongly supported by both ethical principles and legal precedents. The primary ethical principle supporting the withdrawal of life-sustaining therapies is respect for autonomy [46]. In a series of cases addressing withdrawal of life-sustaining therapies, the US courts have ruled that the right to make decisions about medical treatments is both a common law (derived from court decisions) right based on bodily integrity and self-determination and a constitutional right based on privacy and liberty [47, 48]. A patient has the right to refuse any treatment, even if the treatment prolongs life and death would follow a decision not to use it [49]. US Supreme Court decisions have made a clear distinction between withdrawing life-sustaining treatments and assisted suicide and euthanasia. In the case of *Vacco v. Quill* [50], Chief Justice Rehnquist wrote, "The distinction comports with fundamental legal principles of causation and intent. First, when a patient refuses life-sustaining medical treatment, he dies from an underlying fatal disease or pathology; but if a patient ingests lethal medication prescribed by a physician, he is killed by that medication... [In *Cruzan*] our assumption of a right to refuse treatment was grounded not…on the proposition that patients have a…right to hasten death, but on well established, traditional rights to bodily integrity and freedom from unwanted touching." Further, courts have ruled that there is no legal difference between withdrawing an ongoing treatment and not starting in the first place. Granting requests to withdraw life-sustaining treatments from patients, who do not want them, is respecting a right to be left alone and to die naturally of the underlying disease, a legally protected right based on the right to privacy. This has been phrased "a right to decide how to live the rest of one's life."

The Supreme Court has not specifically addressed the question of PM or ICD deactivation. However, the prior rulings did not focus on the specific therapy under question, but rather on "life-sustaining therapies." The law applies to the person, and informed consent is a right of the patient—it is not specific to any one medical intervention [49, 51–53].Thus, because cardiac implanted electronic devices deliver life-sustaining therapies, discontinuation of these therapies is clearly addressed by the Supreme Court precedents upholding the right to discontinue life-sustaining treatment—"Procedures don't have rights, patients do." Finally, these rights extend to patients who lack decision-making capacity, through previously expressed statements (e.g., advance directive) and surrogate decision-makers [51, 54, 55].

Importance of Early, Proactive Communication

Timely and effective communication is critical to prevent painful shocks in patients nearing the end of their lives. When first reported in 2004, few patients had discussed deactivation with their physicians prior to death [41].Ten and 15 years later, many patients remain unaware of the possibility of deactivation [31]. As evidenced by a survey in 2018, a third of patients remain insufficiently aware of ICD deactivation [33]. Similarly, mention of an ICD in an advance directive (AD) was rare in 2006 and 2007 [56, 57], and while the use of ADs is increasing, the proportion of ICD patients completing these remains under 50% [58]. Discussions of patients' goals for their medical care as illness advances have been shown to improve quality of life for these patients [59]. Patients and their families want these interactions with their physicians [60, 61], yet they happen too rarely [41, 45].

Not only is it ethically permissible to discuss with patients their wishes for their care at the end of life, but it is also an ethical imperative to do so. The first principle of medical ethics is autonomy [46], which includes the rights of a patient to self-determination and the duty of clinicians to respect the patient's wishes. Autonomy is maximized when patients understand the nature of their disease and all the options for treatment. These discussions should occur throughout the course of a patient's illness, and the early implementation of an advance directive will maximize a patient's self-determination should he or she become no longer capable of decision-making, as well as decreasing ethical dilemmas and burden on caregiver surrogate decision-makers [45].

However, proactive communication by physicians regarding the option of ICD deactivation remains inadequate. Many barriers to these discussions have been identified [62, 63]. Clinicians report feelings that patients may not be "ready" or that such a discussion will destroy hope or general discomfort.

Clinicians must take a proactive role in discussions about the option of deactivation in the context of the patient's goals for care. These conversations should include a discussion of quality of life, functional status, perceptions of dignity, and both current and potential future symptoms, as each of these elements can influence how patients set goals for their health care [45]. These conversations should continue over the course of the patient's illness. As illness progresses, patient preferences for outcomes and the level of burden acceptable to a patient may change [64, 65]. Advanced care planning conversations improve outcomes for both patients and their families [59], as patients with ICDs who engage in advance care planning are less likely to experience shocks while dying because ICD deactivation has occurred [66]. Studies show that patients and families desire conversations about end-of-life care [60, 61, 67].

Palliative care consultation can also play a role [45, 68]. The goal of palliative care is to relieve suffering and improve quality of life for patients with advanced disease, and palliative care can be simultaneous with life-prolonging care [69]. Palliative care clinicians are expert at discussing values and preferences. Palliative care consultation has been associated with increased use of ADs in patients with ICDs [58]. However, cardiologists cannot abdicate responsibility for discussion with patients. As described by Quill, an overreliance on palliative care specialists may undermine the therapeutic relationship and further fragment care, and he has advocated a "sustainable model for palliative care" as involving both general physicians and palliative specialists [70].

Ongoing efforts may improve communication around ICD deactivation. An ongoing multicenter randomized trial, "Working to Improve Discussions About Defibrillator Management" (WISDOM), is currently evaluating the efficacy of a communication intervention to increase conversations about advance care planning between heart failure clinicians and advanced heart failure patients with ICDs [71], with the primary endpoint of a goals-of-care conversation between patients and clinicians and secondary endpoints ICD deactivation and patient and bereaved satisfaction with care. Incorporation of advanced care planning into the consent process at the time of implant has been suggested [72]. Training of cardiologists in communication around goals of care is critical [63, 73].

References

1. Ahmad M, L B, Roelke M, Bernstein AD, Parsonnet V. Patients' attitudes toward implanted defibrillator shocks. PACE. 2000;23:934–8.
2. Schron E, Exner D, Yao Q, Jenkins L, Steinberg J, Cook J, Kutalek S, Friedman P, Bubien R, Page R, Powell J. Quality of life in the antiarrhythmics versus implantable defibrillators. Circulation. 2002;105:589–94.

3. De Roo ML, van der Steen JT, Galindo Garre F, Van Den Noortgate N, Onwuteaka-Philipsen BD, Deliens L, Francke AL, Euro I. When do people with dementia die peacefully? An analysis of data collected prospectively in long-term care settings. Palliat Med. 2014;28:210–9.
4. Epstein AE, DiMarco JP, Ellenbogen KA, et al. ACC/AHA/HRS 2008 guidelines for device-based therapy of cardiac rhythm abnormalities: a report of the American College of Cardiology/ American Heart Association Task Force on Practice Guidelines (Writing Committee to Revise the ACC/AHA/NASPE 2002 Guideline Update for Implantation of Cardiac Pacemakers and Antiarrhythmia Devices): developed in collaboration with the American Association for Thoracic Surgery and Society of Thoracic Surgeons. Circulation. 2008;117:e350–408.
5. Al-Khatib SM, Stevenson WG, Ackerman MJ, et al. 2017 AHA/ACC/HRS guideline for management of patients with ventricular arrhythmias and the prevention of sudden cardiac death: a report of the American College of Cardiology/American Heart Association Task Force on Clinical Practice Guidelines and the Heart Rhythm Society. Heart Rhythm. 2017;15:e73–e189.
6. Beauregard L. Ethics in electrophysiology: a complaint from palliative care. PACE. 2010;33:226–7.
7. Kobza R, Erne P. End of life decisions in patients with malignant tumors. PACE. 2007;30:845–9.
8. AMA Council on Ethical and Judicial Affairs. AMA 2008–2009. Code of Medical Ethics: Current Opinions and Annotations. 2008–2009 ed. Chicago: AMA Press; 2010.
9. Kramer DB, Matlock DD, Buxton AE, et al. Implantable cardioverter-defibrillator use in older adults: proceedings of a Hartford change AGEnts symposium. Circ Cardiovasc Qual Outcomes. 2015;8:437–46.
10. Heidenreich PA, Tsai V. Is anyone too old for an implantable cardioverter-defibrillator? Circ Cardiovasc Qual Outcomes. 2009;2(1):6–8.
11. Santangeli P, Di Biase L, Dello Russo A, Casella M, Bartoletti S, Santarelli P, Pelargonio G, Natale A. Meta-analysis: age and effectiveness of prophylactic implantable cardioverter-defibrillators. Ann Intern Med. 2010;153:592–9.
12. Hess PL, Al-Khatib SM, Han JY, et al. Survival benefit of the primary prevention implantable cardioverter-defibrillator among older patients: does age matter? An analysis of pooled data from 5 clinical trials. Circ Cardiovasc Qual Outcomes. 2015;8:179–86.
13. Yung D, Birnie D, Dorian P, Healey JS, Simpson CS, Crystal E, Krahn AD, Khaykin Y, Cameron D, Chen Z, Lee DS. Survival after implantable cardioverter-defibrillator implantation in the elderly. Circulation. 2013;127(24):2383–92.
14. Groeneveld PW, Farmer SA, Suh JJ, Matta MA, Yang F. Outcomes and costs of implantable cardioverter-defibrillators for primary prevention of sudden cardiac death among the elderly. Heart Rhythm. 2008;5:646–53.
15. Hernandez AF, Fonarow GC, Hammill BG, Al-Khatib SM, Yancy CW, O'Connor CM, Schulman KA, Peterson ED, Curtis LH. Clinical effectiveness of implantable cardioverter-defibrillators among Medicare beneficiaries with heart failure. Circ Heart Fail. 2010;3:7–13.
16. Huang DT, Sesselberg HW, McNitt S, Noyes K, Andrews ML, Hall WJ, Dick A, Daubert JP, Zareba W, Moss AJ, Group M-IR. Improved survival associated with prophylactic implantable defibrillators in elderly patients with prior myocardial infarction and depressed ventricular function: a MADIT-II substudy. J Cardiovasc Electrophysiol. 2007;18:833–8.
17. Sears SF, Lewis TS, Kuhl EA, Conti JB. Predictors of quality of life in patients with implantable cardioverter defibrillators. Psychosomatics. 2005;46:451–7.
18. Tsai V, Goldstein MK, Hsia HH, Wang Y, Curtis J, Heidenreich PA. Influence of age on perioperative complications among patients undergoing implantable cardioverter-defibrillators for primary prevention in the United States. Circ Cardiovasc Qual Outcomes. 2011;4(5):549–56.
19. Mandawat A, Curtis JP, Mandawat A, Njike VY, Lampert R. Safety of pacemaker implantation in nonagenarians: an analysis of the healthcare cost and utilization project-nationwide inpatient sample. Circulation. 2013;127:1453–65.. 1465e1451-1452
20. Green AR, Leff B, Wang Y, Spatz ES, Masoudi FA, Peterson PN, Daugherty SL, Matlock DD. Geriatric conditions in patients undergoing defibrillator implantation for prevention of sudden cardiac death: Prevalence and impact on mortality. Circ Cardiovasc Qual Outcomes. 2016;9:23–30.

21. Chan PS, Nallamothu BK, Spertus JA, Masoudi FA, Bartone C, Kereiakes DJ, Chow T. Impact of age and medical comorbidity on the effectiveness of implantable cardioverter-defibrillators for primary prevention. Circ Cardiovasc Qual Outcomes. 2009;2:16–24.
22. Husebo BS, Achterberg W, Flo E. Identifying and managing pain in people with Alzheimer's disease and other types of dementia: a systematic review. CNS Drugs. 2016;30:481–97.
23. Lampert R, Soufer R, McPherson CA, Batsford WP, Tirado S, Earley C, Goldberg A, Shusterman V. Implantable cardioverter-defibrillator shocks increase T-wave alternans. J Cardiovasc Electrophysiol. 2007;18:512–7.
24. Mitchell SL, Miller SC, Teno JM, Kiely DK, Davis RB, Shaffer ML. Prediction of 6-month survival of nursing home residents with advanced dementia using ADEPT vs hospice eligibility guidelines. JAMA. 2010;304:1929–35.
25. Wolfson C, Wolfson DB, Asgharian M, M'Lan CE, Ostbye T, Rockwood K, Hogan DB, Clinical Progression of Dementia Study G. A reevaluation of the duration of survival after the onset of dementia. N Engl J Med. 2001;344:1111–6.
26. Barry MJ, Edgman-Levitan S. Shared decision making — the pinnacle of patient-centered care. N Engl J Med. 2012;366:780–1.
27. Mitchell SL, Teno JM, Kiely DK, Shaffer ML, Jones RN, Prigerson HG, Volicer L, Givens JL, Hamel MB. The clinical course of advanced dementia. N Engl J Med. 2009;361:1529–38.
28. Eiser AR, Kirkpatrick JN, Patton KK, McLain E, Dougherty CM, Beattie JM. Putting the "informed" in the informed consent process for implantable cardioverter-defibrillators: addressing the needs of the elderly patient. Pace-Pacing Clin Electrophysiol. 2018;41:312–20.
29. Yancy CW, Jessup M, Bozkurt B, et al. 2013 ACCF/AHA guideline for the management of heart failure: executive summary: a report of the American College of Cardiology Foundation/American Heart Association Task Force on practice guidelines. Circulation. 2013;128:1810–52.
30. Centers for Medicare and Medicaid Services. Decision memo for implantable cardioverter defibrillators (CAG-00157R4). 2018.; https://www.cms.gov/medicare-coverage-database/details/nca-decision-memo.aspx?NCAId=288.
31. Lewis KB, Stacey D, Matlock DD. Making decisions about implantable cardioverter-defibrillators from implantation to end of life: an integrative review of patients' perspectives. Patient. 2014;7:243–60.
32. Yuhas J, Mattocks K, Gravelin L, Remetz M, Foley J, Fazio R, Lampert R. Patients' attitudes and perceptions of implantable cardioverter-defibrillators: potential barriers to appropriate primary prophylaxis. Pacing Clin Electrophysiol. 2012;35:1179–87.
33. McEvedy SM, Cameron J, Lugg E, et al. Implantable cardioverter defibrillator knowledge and end-of-life device deactivation: a cross-sectional survey. Palliat Med. 2018;32:156–63.
34. Matlock DD, Nowels CT, Masoudi FA, Sauer WH, Bekelman DB, Main DS, Kutner JS. Patient and cardiologist perceptions on decision making for implantable cardioverter-defibrillators: a qualitative study. Pacing Clin Electrophysiol. 2011;34:1634–44.
35. Matlock DD, Jones J, Nowels CT, Jenkins A, Allen LA, Kutner JS. Evidence of cognitive bias in decision making around implantable-cardioverter defibrillators: a qualitative framework analysis. J Card Fail. 2017;23:794–9.
36. Green AR, Jenkins A, Masoudi FA, Magid DJ, Kutner JS, Leff B, Matlock DD. Decision-making experiences of patients with implantable cardioverter defibrillators. Pacing Clin Electrophysiol. 2016;39:1061–9.
37. Stacey D, Légaré F, Lewis K, Barry MJ, Bennett CL, Eden KB, Holmes-Rovner M, Llewellyn-Thomas H, Lyddiatt A, Thomson R, L Trevena. Decision aids to help people who are facing health treatment or screening decisions. Cochran Revi 2017.; https://www.cochrane.org/CD001431/COMMUN_decision-aids-help-people-who-are-facing-health-treatment-or-screening-decisions.
38. Caverly TJ, Al-Khatib SM, Kutner JS, Masoudi FA, Matlock DD. Patient preference in the decision to place implantable cardioverter-defibrillators. Arch Intern Med. 2012;172:1104–5.
39. Nambisan V, Chao D. Death and defibrillation: a shocking experience. Palliat Med. 2004;18:482–3.

40. Looi YC. And it can go on and on and on. J Pain Symptom Manag. 2006;31:1–2.
41. Goldstein NE, Lampert R, Bradley E, Lynn J, Krumholz HM. Management of Implantable cardioverter defibrillators in end-of-life care. Ann Intern Med. 2004;141:835–8.
42. Kinch Westerdahl A, Sjöblom J, Mattiasson A, Rosenqvist M, Frykman V. Implantable defibrillator therapy before death – high risk for painful shocks at end of life. Circulation. 2014;129(4):422–9.
43. Stewart GC, Weintraub JR, Pratibhu PP, et al. Patient expectations from implantable defibrillators to prevent death in heart failure. J Cardiac Fail. 2010;16:106–13.
44. Dodson JA, Fried TR, Van Ness PH, Goldstein N, Lampert R. Patient preferences for deactivation of implantable cardioverter defibrillators. JAMA Intern Med. 2013;173:377–9.
45. Lampert R, Hayes DL, Annas GJ, et al. HRS expert consensus statement on the management of Cardiovascular Implantable Electronic Devices (CIEDs) in patients nearing end of life or requesting withdrawal of therapy. Heart Rhythm. 2010;7:1008–26.
46. Beauchamp TL. Principles of biomedical ethics. 6th ed. New York: Oxford University Press; 2009.
47. Quinlan IR. 70 N.J. 10, 355 A.2d 647 New Jersey Supreme Court 1976.
48. Cruzan vs Director Missouri Department of Health. 497 U.S. 261 88–1503. 1990.
49. Annas GJ. The rights of patients: the authoritative ACLU guide to the rights of patients. 3rd ed. New York: New York University Press; 2004.
50. Vacco v Quill. [521 U.S. 793, 95–1858. Supreme Court of the United States. 1997.
51. Annas GJ. "Culture of life" politics at the bedside--the case of Terri Schiavo. N Engl J Med. 2005;352:1710–5.
52. Burt RA. Death is that man taking names. Berkeley: University of California Press; 2002.
53. Schneider C. The practice of autonomy: patients, doctors, and medical decisions. New York: Oxford University Press; 1998.
54. Quill TE, Barold SS, Sussman BL. Discontinuing an implantable cardioverter defibrillator as a life-sustaining treatment. Am J Cardiol. 1994;74:205–7.
55. Wiegand DL, Kalowes PG. Withdrawal of cardiac medications and devices. AACN Adv Crit Care. 2007;18:415–25.
56. Berger JT, Gorski M, Cohen T. Advance health planning and treatment preferences among recipients of implantable cardioverter defibrillators: an exploratory study. J Clin Ethics. 2006;17:72–8.
57. Tajouri TH, Ottenberg AL, Hayes DL, Mueller PS. The use of advance directives among patients with implantable cardioverter defibrillators. Pacing Clin Electrophysiol. 2012;35:567–73.
58. Merchant FM, Binney Z, Patel A, Li J, Peddareddy LP, El-Chami MF, Leon AR, Quest T. Prevalence, Predictors and outcomes of advance directives in implantable cardioverter defibrillator recipients. Heart Rhythm. 2017;14(6):830–6.
59. Wright AA, Zhang B, Ray A, Mack JW, Trice E, Balboni T, Mitchell SL, Jackson VA, Block SD, Maciejewski PK, Prigerson HG. Associations between end-of-life discussions, patient mental health, medical care near death, and caregiver bereavement adjustment. JAMA. 2008;300:1665–73.
60. Fried TR, O'Leary JR. Using the experiences of bereaved caregivers to inform patient- and caregiver-centered advance care planning. J Gen Intern Med. 2008;23:1602–7.
61. Singer PA, Martin DK, Kelner M. Quality end-of-life care: patients' perspectives. JAMA. 1999;281:163–8.
62. Goldstein NE, Mehta D, Teitelbaum E, Bradley EH, Morrison RS. "It's like crossing a bridge" complexities preventing physicians from discussing deactivation of implantable defibrillators at the end of life. J Gen Intern Med. 2008;1:2–6.
63. Dunlay SM, Strand JJ. How to discuss goals of care with patients. Trends Cardiovasc Med. 2016;26:36–43.
64. Fried TR, Bradley EH, Towle VR, Allore H. Understanding the treatment preferences of seriously ill patients. N Engl J Med. 2002;346:1061–6.

65. Fried TR, Byers AL, Gallo WT, Van Ness PH, Towle VR, O'Leary JR, Dubin JA. Prospective study of health status preferences and changes in preferences over time in older adults. Arch Intern Med. 2006;166:890–5.
66. Lewis WR, Luebke DL, Johnson NJ, Harrington MD, Costantini O, Aulisio MP. Withdrawing implantable defibrillator shock therapy in terminally ill patients. Am J Med. 2006;119:892–6.
67. Nicolasora N, Pannala R, Mountantonakis S, Shanmugam B, DeGirolamo A, Amoateng-Adjepong Y, Manthous CA. If asked, hospitalized patients will choose whether to receive life-sustaining therapies. J Hosp Med. 2006;1:161–7.
68. Buchhalter LC, Ottenberg AL, Webster TL, Swetz KM, Hayes DL, Mueller PS. Features and outcomes of patients who underwent cardiac device deactivation. JAMA Intern Med. 2014;174:80–5.
69. Morrison RS, Meier DE. Clinical practice. Palliative care. N Engl J Med. 2004;350:2582–90.
70. Quill TE, Abernethy AP. Generalist plus specialist palliative care – creating a more sustainable model. N Engl J Med. 2013;368:1173–5.
71. Goldstein NE, Kalman J, Kutner JS, Fromme EK, Hutchinson MD, Lipman HI, Matlock DD, Swetz KM, Lampert R, Herasme O, Morrison RS. A study to improve communications between clinicians and patients with advanced heart failure: methods and challenges behind the working to improve discussions about defibrillator management trial. J Pain Symptom Manag. 2014;48:1236–46.
72. Kirkpatrick JN, Hauptman PJ, Goodlin SJ. Bundling informed consent and advance care planning in chronic cardiovascular disease we need to talk. JAMA Intern Med. Jan 2015;175:5–6.
73. Butler K, Puri S. Deathbed shock causes and cures. JAMA Intern Med. 2014;174:88–9.

Index

© Springer Nature Switzerland AG 2019
J. S. Steinberg, A. E. Epstein (eds.), *Clinical Controversies in Device Therapy
for Cardiac Arrhythmias*, https://doi.org/10.1007/978-3-030-22882-8

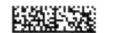